Welcome to my story. It is about a journey into a realm of anxiety and depression. If you are currently suffering from these conditions, you can understand how difficult it can be to simply get up in the morning and try to live a normal life.

The truth is that there are days when you just can't, and it's hard to make it through the day, but you try your hardest to do so. You yearn so hard to live a normal life, but it's like walking around with a boulder around your neck.

It's been a long journey for me, and that is why I wanted to share the information in this book. I want others who are experiencing anxiety and depression to know that they are not alone and that they don't have to suffer in silence. If you are currently going through this situation, then I want you to know that there is nothing wrong with you.

If anything, you are very brave and strong!

Merely by getting up in the morning, you have faced and defeated one of the biggest monsters you will ever face in your life.

If you are reading this because you want to help someone going through anxiety and depression, I want you to know that just being there for them is the best thing you can do. Your loved ones may not always express appreciation, but believe me, they do. As a matter of fact, you might be the only thing holding them together.

So, here is my story. I hope it helps you to find answers, especially when it seems like everything is just one giant mess.

The reason for the repetition of certain aspects of this writing is to emphasize their importance and to serve as reminders of the calamity and anguish that those like me who suffered and may still suffer from anxiety and depression.

Magdy Hussein, PhD.

Table of Contents

Part I "The Free Fall"

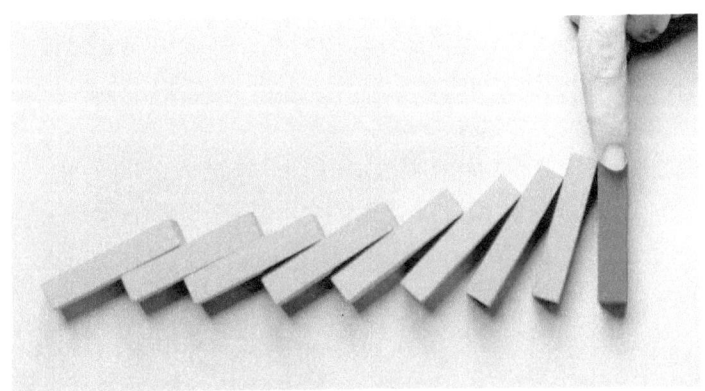

Chapter 1: The Horrifying Flight

I didn't always feel like this.

You could say I was one lucky person, married to a beautiful wife, had awesome children, a great job, and had a decent income.

I was just like everyone else. I thought about the weekend, going on vacation, and hanging out with my family. I was respected and appreciated at work. My boss was a bit tough and demanding, but super cool. He was the kind of boss you like working for.

I was in my late thirties and staring down at a settled and meaningful job that would take me to retirement. People who knew me back then would have said that I had figured everything out. I am a people-oriented person who likes to make sense of what I am doing, so I can go home with a peaceful conscious.

There was no reason why I couldn't devour the entire world!

Looking back on things, I realized that I was working quite hard. I was averaging about eight to ten hours at the office every day. I usually took work home with me just so I could catch up with everything. There were times I would go to bed early and wake up early or stay up late just to get ahead.

I was committed to being the best that I could be. But then again, that was also beginning to affect me. I wasn't as cheerful as I was, and I admit, there were a few occasions when I was very stressed out. But I always managed to work things out, eat well, and enjoy an active social life. I worked hard during the week so that I could enjoy my weekends without having to worry about work piling up on me.

One of the most important parts of my job was to visit customers on-site. I needed to make personal visits so that I could serve them more effectively. This part of my job meant frequent air flights. That also meant a lot of time spent at airports and working on airplanes. I didn't mind those flights because it was a time when I could disconnect or perhaps catch up on some work.

I was used to frequent air flights. I would make several each month. Sometimes, it would be several flights a week. Still, it didn't get to me, even though I must admit that there were times when flying did irritate me. I suppose it was just the stress from being on the move all the time.

The day things changed…

I was headed to St. John's, Canada, to visit a customer. This was a bit of a tough flight, as I had several connections before my destination. It wasn't that bad, but multiple connections can be a hassle.

The trip to St. John's was uneventful. As I said, it was long with multiple connections. I had a good meeting with my customer, so it was quite successful. I was feeling good about myself. It seemed like things were going well.

Did I jinx myself?

Not likely…

Anyway, I had a three-leg flight from St. John's to San Jose, California. I didn't think much of it. I just felt it was a bit of a hassle, but it was the best flight I could get. My first flight took me from St. John's to Montreal. That is where my life would change forever.

Mid-air, the small aircraft I was in experienced some serious turbulence. Had it been a large airplane like a 747, it might not have been that bad. But since this was a small aircraft, the kind that only seats around 50 people, the turbulence rocked the plane like it was a child's toy.

Panic ensued.

Everyone aboard the plane was caught completely unawares. The bump was so violent that the foodservice tray flew into the pilot's cabin. One of the crew was knocked down while the others managed to grab on.

All I could do was close my eyes and grab the seat handles. Although I couldn't see my knuckles, I was certain that they had turned white. I tried to grab as hard as I could, and I barely managed to open my eyes. As I looked around, I could see the other passengers holding on for dear life as well. I could tell they were just as terrified as I was. So, I just closed my eyes even tighter.

I think I started to pray, but then I suddenly got flashes of my life, 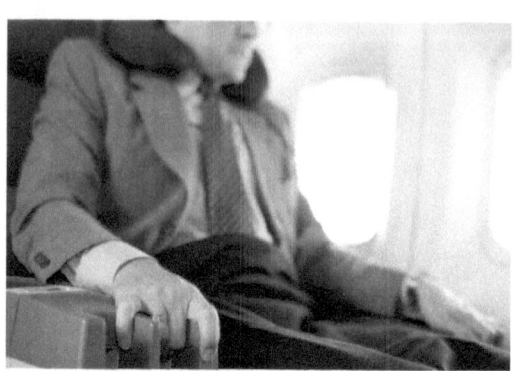 and I felt agony. It felt like I couldn't breathe. The turbulence was so intense that I felt my body go numb. Instantly, I got flashes of the airplane hitting a mountain or something else. I could imagine seeing the fuselage being ripped apart and people flying out into the sky to their demise. I could picture the wreckage and all of those dead bodies on the ground. The carnage was indescribable.

I had never really feared for my life, for I had never really been in a situation in which I thought I would surely die.

Well, as is said, there is always a first time. I suppose that the turbulence only lasted a few moments. A couple of minutes tops, but it seemed like an eternity. Everyone was visibly shaken. People were crying, both men and women. I could hear people gasping for air.
But as for the airplane, no damage occurred. It was as if nothing had happened at all.

Oh, but something did happen. Something happened, alright!

Had this been a single flight, I guess I might have been able to recover. But when I realized I still had two more flights to catch before reaching California, I almost panicked. I couldn't bear to think that something like that would ever happen again.

How would you have felt after such a horrendous experience?

I could hear the other passengers chatter as we got off the airplane. They were thanking their lucky stars to be alive, but at the same time, they were distraught after what had happened.

I was literally emotionally shattered. I thought about just sitting in the airport and not getting back on the airplane. By the way, passengers get in an airplane and not on it, but I managed to build up the courage to make my next flight.

By all measures, the next two flights were uneventful. I went through security, got on the airplane, got off the airplane, and then in it again. I arrived in California in one piece. Well, perhaps my body was in one piece, but my mind was in a million fragments.

Things didn't get any better. I was still nervous and anxious. I didn't have too much trouble going about my usual business. But I knew something was wrong.

Everything became worse a few days later. I had to fly to New York City to meet with my family. We had booked a vacation there months earlier. It should have been a great time, but I didn't enjoy a minute of it. The flight to New York was excruciating. I curled up in my seat during the entire flight. During the trip, I tried my best to enjoy the flight, but I felt like a soulless automaton. I was as if I were just a robot moving about. The flight back was also torture.

I just couldn't stop thinking about the airplane crashing to the ground. I couldn't get these images of death, destruction, and annihilation out of my mind.

I knew that this wasn't normal. But I just couldn't understand what was going on…

The new abnormal…
After returning home, I went about my usual routine. I tried to focus on work. I was certain that work would get my mind off what had happened. I knew that if I buckled down, I would get through it. Boy, was I wrong?

Anxiety attacks became the norm. At the time, I didn't know they were anxiety attacks. All I knew was that I couldn't breathe, my chest was pounding, and my body pulsated. I thought I was having a heart attack. I went to a hospital, Emergency Room (ER) several times. Each time I went, my tests were fine, and even a visit to a cardiologist proved that there was nothing physically wrong with me.

A few weeks later, my company scheduled a trip for me to Sweden. I did not reveal my feelings of anxiety and decided to push through it.

That was when I really broke down. I made it to Heathrow Airport in England with an ambulance waiting for me. I was taken to a hospital to ensure that I had not suffered a heart attack. I managed to make my flight to Sweden the next day, and I managed to get through with my tasks and flew back home.

I was in a terrible condition. The anxiety attacks just kept getting worse and worse. I was eventually referred to a psychiatrist. After multiple evaluations, I was diagnosed with major depression.

My company grounded me. I could no longer travel by air. The medications that were prescribed for me helped me feel better by numbing the pain.

Ultimately, I had to take a disability leave of absence and seek treatment.

Chapter 2: The Confusion

I suppose having depression really isn't the worst part of my situation. I mean, it's like you're not living your own life. Thanks to the medications, I felt like I was permanently floating on a cloud. In a way, they helped because they allowed me to calm down many of the negative, nagging feelings and thoughts that I had. These thoughts gnawed at me over and over again.

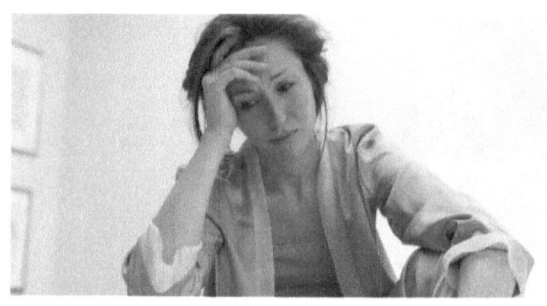

It's tough to deal with those kinds of thoughts. There are times when you feel perfectly fine. Thankfully, it's been a good day. You manage to get things done, maybe even go out with friends. It's a great feeling to get out of bed, go about your usual business, and see progress, but eventually the relief that I had felt from the prescribed medications began to diminish.

And then, wham! It's like you're hit with a sledgehammer. All of those negative thoughts come rushing to your mind. You start thinking about the worst things that could happen. Now, I don't mean scary stuff like what you see on TV. Horror movies are kiddie time compared to the sheer terror that you feel during an anxiety attack.

Most of the time, my mind would race. It was a flood of thoughts, image after image of the most incredibly terrifying mental reflections. Sometimes, it would be flashbacks of the ill-fated airplane ride. Other times, it would be just random things.

Do you know what the worst part was? It was that there wasn't a specific trigger. It wasn't like I was going to the airport and then going to Berserk. It was literally anything that could trigger these attacks. I couldn't determine what caused them. It was like they could happen at any time and for any reason.

I felt as though I was going insane!

I honestly tried to figure things out. I tried to make sense of what was happening, but to no avail. There was nothing that I could pinpoint. I thought that if I could just figure out what it was that was affecting me so adversely, I could then go back to being myself.

Nothing.

Just isolation and fear. I ended up staying at home most of the time. I stopped going out because I was terrified of losing it in public. As a result, my physical appearance started to be affected. I gained weight and quickly went out of shape. I hardly looked my best.

Then the lack of sleep began to take its toll on me. I couldn't sleep through the night. I would wake up every two hours, usually in a panic and for no reason in particular. I had frequent nightmares. I usually woke up fearing that I was going to have an anxiety attack, and sure enough, I would.

This meant frequent trips to the ER.
I felt as if my life was no longer mine. It was practically meaningless. My emotional condition was in ruins. It was as if a nuclear bomb had been dropped on my emotional and physical well-being. All the doctors could do was to prescribe more and more medications.

But nothing seemed to work.

It was like the more medications that I took, the worse I got. Explanations from doctors did not suffice. They couldn't tell me what was wrong. I craved, I yearned to know what was afflicting me. I just needed to know what was wrong with me. But no answers. Just more and more medications.

As I said, the medications helped a bit. They tend to take the edge off at times. But the downside to it is that you feel numb. You feel nothing at all. It's like you're this half-human, half-machine creation.

That's no way to live a life with such an experience. How can it be life if you can't think straight? How can you enjoy life when you don't have any feelings? Sure, the attacks may not be as often or as severe, but they don't go away completely. So, what's the point of taking the medications if you still get the attacks?

I was nothing more than a lab rat for the pharmaceutical companies.

It felt like doctors were just trying random ideas to see what worked. And when something didn't work, they would try something else. And when that didn't work, they would try something else again. Eventually, they ran out of ideas.

How is that possible?

How can it be that doctors, who are trained professionals, can't figure out what's wrong with you?

In the end, the questions that ravaged my brain were worse than the memories of the air flight. Even though I had realized that the flight was the catalyst for all of this, I was desperate to know why this was happening to me. I was absolutely going up the wall, trying to figure things out.

You see, the thing is that anxiety and depression create a negative feedback loop. They feed one another. Generally, anxiety hits first. It starts off with panic attacks, but they temporarily go away. You manage to deal with them. But then they get worse and worse.

Anxiety eventually leads to depression. Now, most people believe depression is about being sad. They think that depression is about crying all the time. That's only a part of it. Depression is about losing the will to live. It's about not having any reason to get up in the morning. It's about questioning why you are even on this Earth.

So, when those dark, nasty thoughts kick in, that triggers anxiety, which then triggers an attack.

It's a negative feedback loop. The greater the depression, the greater the attacks. The greater the attacks, the greater the depression. It just keeps getting worse and worse. No matter how hard you try to make it work, you just can't. There are days when you run out of steam. You run out of the will to live. You don't have any strength left in you.

Depression is a soul-sucking force. It's like having your energy drained by an astronomical black hole. The force is so strong that it is inescapable. There seems to be no way out of it.

Once it sucks you in, you feel that you can't get out.

As the days passed, my madness grew stronger. I couldn't understand why this was happening to me. The more I wanted to make sense of it all, the fewer answers I could come up with. I tried desperately to search for answers.

Often, when I tried an online search, I would come away feeling shattered. There was just so much information to take in. It was too much for my brain to process and absorb. I mean, I know I'm smart, but I just couldn't process all that information. It was too much for me to handle.

I read some fascinating stories about people who recovered from major depression. They really seemed inspiring, but they weren't me. These stories didn't sound like what I was going through. Most stories dealt with the loss of a loved one or being the victim of abuse.

But that wasn't me!

I mean, have you ever tried to figure out a puzzle that you just couldn't make heads or tails of?

Getting a grip on my life was just like that. I couldn't put the pieces together. Well, that was assuming the pieces were there to begin with. No matter how hard I tried, I just couldn't come up with answers.

To make matters worse, every time I tried to talk about my feelings with someone, I couldn't talk for more than a few minutes. All of the emotions that came rushing at me all at once were simply too much to bear. It's like trying to stop a tidal wave. No force on Earth can stop such an immense blast of emotions. No matter what you do, all you can hope for is to brace yourself for the impact. In fact, that's what I did every time I thought about that ill-fated air flight.

They say that time heals all wounds. Well, I suppose it does heal wounds. But does time really heal a shattered soul?

That's a question that I often ponder. I couldn't imagine how people could live with depression for years and years. It seems incredible to think that there are people who can carry on with their lives as if nothing had happened.

But then again, it takes a great deal of courage to admit you need help, but I was never ashamed of admitting that I needed help, and it was just so frustrating to see that I wasn't getting it. I just wanted to rid myself of this unbearable burden. But the harder I tried, the more it weighed down on me.

At least the good days were a welcome reprieve. However, the bad days were the worst. It took me a while to recover from those days. Still, I didn't want to give up. I thought about quitting many times. But I'm not a quitter. I'm a fighter, so I needed to figure something out. Something had to give. The medications weren't working. There had to be a solution somewhere. I was certain that somehow, I was going to figure it out.

Chapter 3: The Imminent Death

One of the thoughts that I just couldn't get out of my mind was "this is it!" Every time I had a panic attack, I felt like this was the near-fatal one. I felt like I was going to literally die!

Some folks had told me that I'm just overreacting when I mentioned my symptoms, but these are people who have never gone through my experiences. When you go through the agony that accompanies a panic and an anxiety attack, you can understand how terrifying it can be.

Mainly, a panic attack is like being unable to breathe. No matter how hard you try, you can't catch your breath. This makes things worse because you're already freaked out, and on top of that, you're absolutely frightened by the fact that you can't breathe easily. You begin to fear for your life.

But that's not the worst part.

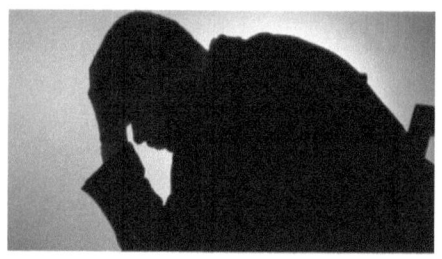

The worst part is the pounding feeling in your chest. You feel like your heart is about to pop out of your chest. Plus, the lack of air makes you dizzy and lightheaded. It's so hard to focus on just one thing: there's the pounding heart, lack of air, lightheadedness, and the dreary and overwhelming feeling of fear.

I remember the first time I went through this. I was completely petrified because I didn't know what was going on. Since that first panic attack, each one just got worse and worse.

Clearly, knowing how bad they can be, you always fear the next one. That alone is enough to set off another attack. If there were only some kind of way that you could predict when the attacks happen, then that would make things easier to handle.

I don't know. Again, every time I had an attack, it just kept feeling worse and worse. Also, bouncing back from an attack kept getting harder and harder. At first, I would just settle down, regain my composure, and try to move on. But I repeat that there were several attacks that landed me in the ER.

Sadly, the trips to the ER became more and more frequent. No matter what I tried to do, the trips to the ER were constant in my life. I would be put on oxygen and given my medications, but nothing seemed to help. Sure, I was comfortable for a while, but as soon as the medications wore off, it was back to square one.

I was just sick and tired of it.

I mean, there's no way to live like this. There were times when I thought it might have been better to just have died on that airplane. That would've spared me from all of this agony that I was going through. It's not that I wanted to die, but seemingly, dying in the airplane crash wouldn't have been as bad as what I was going through.

I also hated the fact that doctors couldn't give me a straight answer. There came a point when I just tried to ignore doctors. What did they know? They weren't going through the same situation as I. So, what could they do? If they could have done something, they would have done it already.

So, I tried to convince myself that things would be alright. I kept telling myself over and over that everything was going to be fine. I didn't want to keep feeling like this anymore. I tried to force my mind to get over what was happening.

There were times when it did work. I figured that if I just ignored the heart attack symptoms, they would somehow go away. I mean, if there wasn't anything physically wrong with me, then it must have all been in my mind, right?

Yeah, guess again…

Sure, such things might be in your mind, but you can't just pull them out like a garden weed. Anxiety is not the type of thing you can just dismiss from your head. As for depression, don't get me started on that! Well, if you must, then depression is like walking around with a dark cloud suspended over your head all the time. You just can't ignore it, no matter how hard you try. Of course, you can dismiss it for a few minutes at a time, but depression has the funniest ways of finding you, and when it catches up to you, let's just say that you feel like you're getting blasted by a rolling boulder.

Since self-talk wasn't getting me anywhere, I needed to find something else that could finally help me get over the hump. I needed to find an alternative to the medications. I needed to make a change that could get my life back to normal.

That's what I wanted more than anything in the world. You could have stacked ten million dollars on a table right in front of me, but that was meaningless to me when compared to getting my life back in order.

I just wanted to go back to the way things were, but with each passing day, it just seemed like that was getting further and further away.

Of all the things I had to go through, the worst part was going to bed every night. I was afraid that it would be my last one on Earth. I was terribly afraid that if I went to sleep, I would not wake up, or that I would have a heart attack, and that would be the end of it.

Just the thought of dying was enough to trigger another attack. It was even worse when I thought about dying in my sleep. I felt so helpless, thinking that no one would be able to rescue me. This led to many sleepless nights. I was already under enough stress, and now I had to contend with more sleep deprivation.

I was physically and mentally exhausted... or you can say "broken".

I wasn't sleeping much anymore. The little sleep I got was terrible. I had attacks coming and going all the time. I couldn't get the dreadful thoughts out of my head. All I could think about was death.

Do you want to know the good part? I didn't want to die!

My life was a complete mess. I couldn't handle it anymore. The mental pain I was going through didn't make life worth living anymore, yet still, I did not want to die. It didn't make any sense, and I didn't know what to do.

One day, I got a flash of light. It was as if someone had flipped on a light switch. I remembered a psychologist friend, K.S. I thought that if anyone could help me, it would be him. I tried everything within my power. The doctors weren't doing much for me. So, why not talk to a psychologist?

I had nothing to lose. What was the worst thing that could happen? At this point, I was willing to try anything. I had hit the lowest possible point I could in my life. Anything, and I really mean *anything*, that could have provided me with some relief was a welcome sight.

I called my psychologist friend, who flew from Arizona to meet with me. We talked about how psychotherapy would provide me with an alternative form of treatment that wasn't drugs or medications. It was just a matter of my being able to talk about what was happening to me.

At first, I was very hesitant to talk about the private things that were affecting me. I wish that I could have just been able to talk and let it all out. However, it turned out to be a process. When you go to therapy, you need to work your way up to what's really bothering you. Then, when you do, you are able to finally come to terms with your biggest fears.

This is where I realized that everything started with that awful air flight. I mean, I knew that flight was the starting point. It was the catalyst, but I hadn't made the conscious discovery that the flight from St. John's to Montreal had triggered so many adverse effects inside of me.

This first stage of the recovery process is what the toughest, and most definitely, the darkest was for me. I was confronted by many demons that I did not know were lurking in the shadows. In fact, as I had previously mentioned, there are times when you feel like you are getting whacked over the head with a sledgehammer.

There were times when I looked at myself in the mirror and somehow couldn't recognize who I was. This part of the journey is about rediscovering who you really are, and it's about finding what you are really made of.

Seriously, sometimes you don't know what to do, how to react, or even what to think. But that's a part of the journey to recovery. Rediscovering yourself is not easy. While it's enlightening in many ways, it can also open up the floodgates to some things you thought were dead and buried.

Part I Closure

It's incredible how much your life can change in a heartbeat. There I was, going about my usual routine, wrapping up another job, when Bam! My whole world turned upside-down.

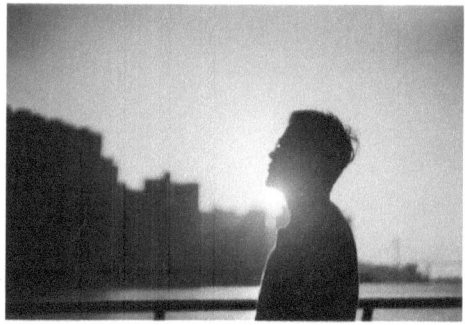

I know that you, the reader, have experienced this at some point or another, or that you know someone who suffers from these experiences. If you are afflicted and think that you have everything figured out, only to realize that you don't. You think that life is perfect when suddenly it isn't.

For me, it was that awful flight. For others, it can be something like getting sick, being in an accident, losing a loved one, or losing everything in a natural disaster.

It really doesn't matter what you are experiencing; all you know is that you are left with an empty feeling inside. It's like a gaping chasm that drags you in completely. No matter how hard you try, you can't seem to get away from it.

That's how I felt.

I felt like the harder I tried, the more that black hole pulled me in. I won't lie; those dark days felt like the end of the world. It felt like the Earth had stopped spinning. Days and nights were simply blurred into a single haze.

But even in that haze, I could see light. It was that light that I tried my hardest to hold on to. That light was the only thing keeping me from losing it altogether.

I know that you must have felt like that many times as well. I can tell you that you must not lose sight of that light. No matter how far away it seems, that light is the only thing that can keep you from giving up.

There were times when I felt I was flipping over rocks trying to find answers to my questions. I was at wits' end trying to get answers. I don't know if I could call it divine inspiration. But when I reached out to my psychologist friend, I knew I was onto something.

To Be Continued...

Part II: "Coming Out of the Dark Hole"

Part I Recap

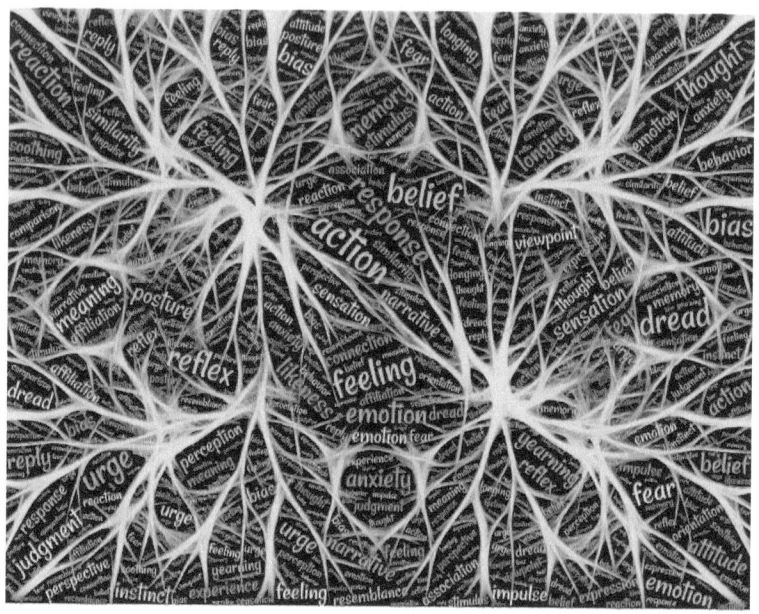

Depression and anxiety are beasts that no person ever wants to face, and yet sometimes we find ourselves there anyway. We find ourselves drowning in our emotions, feeling like getting past them is an impossible task of epic proportions. I found myself there, as I had written about in Part I.

I didn't always feel like this. I was a lucky person with a great family and a great career. Then one day, it all changed. One day was all it took for me to suddenly have my entire world rocked, and it all happened on an airplane. As stated, the airplane literally rocked in turbulence, and while everything was eventually alright and I lived to tell the tale, the truth is that moment defined me. It weighed heavily on who I am as a person, and it influenced

26

everything about me. The person who stepped into that airplane had figuratively died, and I stepped off of it as a changed man. I got out of that airplane as a shell of the person that I was, and everything was different.

I became anxious. I suffered from panic attacks and depression. I couldn't focus any longer. I was confused and felt isolated in that moment. I felt like my mind was racing with many things that I couldn't control, and I was miserable. I couldn't cope with the stress. I needed to somehow get control of my situation, but that was so hard to do when I barely knew "up" from "down", and the ground underneath my feet felt like it had been pulled away.

I rapidly deteriorated. I gained weight. I stopped sleeping. I had panic attacks, and at the end of the day, the only solution was to pump me full of all the medications the doctors could prescribe. I was no longer me, and I was certain that I was going to die. I had panic attacks on a regular basis, and if you've never had one, then you don't understand the sheer terror of such an experience. You don't understand the desperation that I felt when the panic attacks hit. And that brings us to the next part of my story.

If depression itself, the anxiety, and other mental struggles that I faced were a deep hole, then Part II of my journey represents my escape—my ability to get out of the hole and find a way back to the surface. Part II is the part where I was able to answer several questions that I had been pondering in my head. I knew that I had a problem; it was all around me and undeniable. However, I needed to answer my new questions. I'd have to answer the questions about myself and grapple with my own mortality.

As I coped with my depression and anxiety, I asked myself two key questions that defined the next leg of my journey: How soon will I die? If I'm not dying soon, then can I become normal again?

Can I find my way back to living the life that I had before, when I wasn't constantly under assault by my mind? These questions were constantly in my mind. These questions drove me to near insanity; they plagued my waking hours and kept me awake at night.

Ultimately, I found the answers. I eventually learned what I needed to know thanks to four people in my life. My wife was like a coach to me during this time—she was my rock, and I am eternally grateful to her for everything that she has done for me. I'm grateful to my psychologist, who sat with me and helped me work through everything that I needed to know. I'm thankful to my psychiatrist, R.D., whom I saw regularly, and who helped me to cope when I felt like I couldn't. And finally, I'm thankful to my dear friend, SD, who told me of his own survival against depression and anxiety, who gave me hope for the future. I never thought that he had been someone who could have coped with such trauma and grief, and yet he told me that he had, and that he had found his own sense of normalcy. He gave me the answer to my second question and taught me that I didn't have to fear for the future—I just had to move toward it.

This is my story about walking to the other side of depression and anxiety. It's a long and hard journey, but just like any other, it can be broken down step by step, but rather it can be broken down sentence by sentence, and little by little, until I am once again able to identify the truth—that I can do so, and I will be able to achieve that sense of normalcy again. So, for you, my dear reader, take this second part of my story and learn from it. Let this be for you what my dear friend's own story was for me. Look to this as my story of answering my questions, of grappling with my anxiety and depression, and with me coming out on top, more capable and much happier than ever with the ensuing results.

Chapter 4: Touching the Bottom Rock

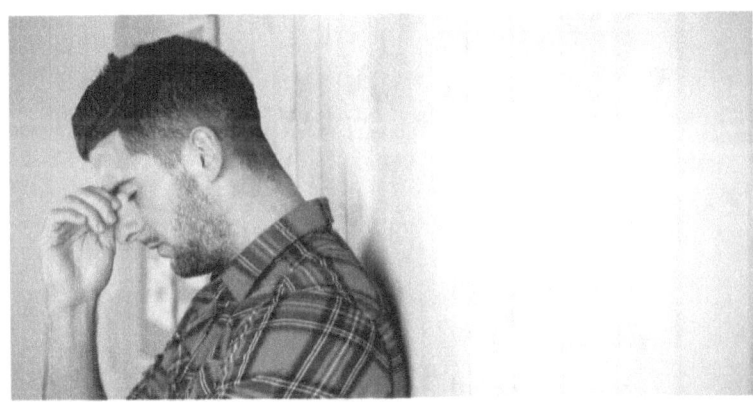

Again, anxiety can be soul-shattering.

One moment, I could be sitting, reading a book as if everything is just fine. I'd be happily turning the pages, ignoring the daily hustle and bustle of my home, with my children and wife moving about me, and I'd be completely immersed in the pages.

The next moment, I felt like I was dying.

I'd realize that my heart is pounding. I'd realize that I couldn't breathe and that every attempt to draw in my breath was harder than the last. I'd feel sheer, unadulterated terror chilling every cell of my being, and I'd believe wholeheartedly that the end was near.

Yes, I knew that I was suffering from anxiety, but that doesn't change the fact that during those moments, all I knew was terror. It became a norm for me. I'd be just fine in one minute, and then panic the next with no rhyme or reason. It felt like it happened completely at random and as if I'd never actually gained control of it.

I don't know if I ever would have gotten control over my anxiety if it weren't for my beautiful wife. She was my rock. My coach. My soft place to fall when everything felt like it was crumbling around me. I owe her everything. I know that if I hadn't had her by my side, I would have gotten worse. I know that if she weren't there with me, I would never have been able to succeed in my recovery.

I remember one time when I was in bed. It was at the end of a long day, and I was beat. I was so ready to fall asleep. I went about my night like normal. I showered, brushed my teeth, changed into my pajamas, and got myself situated in bed. It was welcome respite after the long, hard day, and I knew I'd be asleep before long. My wife was in bed with me—she was reading a book on her side of the bed. I gave her a quick hug and got comfortable.

I felt myself dozing off and surrendered to the sensation, waiting, and just as I was at the brink of consciousness, I started waking again. Suddenly, the same horrific symptoms arose. I was panicking. My heart was racing. I felt like I had pressure on my chest. I was breathing rapidly, and every fiber of my being was absolutely terrified at that time. Every ounce of my body was in full panic mode, and there was nothing that I could do about it.

My wife must have noticed my sudden change in breathing, as I felt her hand gently on my back. She was sitting up, and she pulled me toward her. There, in my panic, I was staring up at my wife, and she looked perfectly calm. I'll never forget that—she seemed like not a single thing was wrong, and she was so great about handling me at that moment.

She asked me a few questions that, at first, sounded strange, but as I calmed down a bit, I realized she had pulled out a Girl Scouts guidebook that had been next to her on the nightstand. First, her hand still on me, she asked me if I was short of breath.

I paused for a moment, thinking about my breathing and focusing on it. Though rapid, my breathing was coming and going with ease. I was no longer short of breath at all, and I answered her, shaking my head in response.

Then she asked the next question. Am I sweating? A quick focus on my body showed that I was just as dry as I had been when I got into bed, and I shook my head no again. I was not sweating.

The final question came just as gently as the last two. She asked me if I had pressure on my chest. I did—it felt like it was constricting me, as if I'd never be able to breathe or function again. I felt like my heart was stuck in my chest, hammering away at my ribcage, and I managed to nod my head.
She nodded her head in understanding at that point and rubbed my back with her hands. She had great news for me at the moment—I probably wasn't having a heart attack because all three of those symptoms would have had to be positive for it to be a heart attack. By default, the next most likely answer was that I was suffering from another anxiety attack. She was so kind and so patient during this time. She asked me what I wanted to do and offered to get my medication to help the attack subside.

My dear and beloved wife was always there for me during these attacks with just as much patience as the ones before, even though she should have been sick of it at some point in time. After all, my constant reliance on her had to have grown old after a while, but she never let on that it was the case. She was just as patient as always.

Now, my attacks weren't always so cleanly resolved. Sometimes, they were so much worse. Sometimes, she'd try her best to talk me through everything and help me feel better, but she wasn't able to do so. It wasn't that she went about things the wrong way. The anxiety had taken too strong a hold on me during those moments. At those times, the best that I could do was go to the emergency room for stabilization, and that was the best course of action for me. It was best for me to be with the professionals sometimes, and they knew how to handle me in order to ensure that I'd be able to go back home comfortably.

No matter what happened, I had my wife there, and I had her support. She was my first lifesaver on this journey, and she made it clear to me that I had to keep going, that I needed to keep on "trucking along". She was the cheerleader that I never realized that I needed on this long trek, and she was always there for me when I needed her.

I owe her more than I will ever be able to put into words. Her kindness, her stolid determination to help me when I felt like I couldn't help myself, and her steadfast nature kept her by my side as I learned to live with my anxiety and depression. She was everything that I ever needed and more, and I can't express my heartfelt gratitude to her.

Of course, she was not the only one at home who helped me, and the other helper that I had in my life actually surprised me when I finally met him.

For years, my kids have always begged me for a pet. Why wouldn't they? They're young kids, and every kid loves animals. At first, I was hesitant—I was busy enough, and I could barely manage to find the time that I needed. I didn't want to stretch myself even thinner by taking care of another pet, so what did I do? I got them a goldfish. They're supposed to be easy to take care of, aren't they? Just dump a few pinches of food in their tank, clean it every now and then, and call it good, right?

We spent some time together getting everything together. We got the tank and filled it up. The kids spent forever agonizing over which goldfish they wanted out of the pet shop tank so that they got just the right one. They picked out some gravel for the tank and a few of those kitschy decorations that you put at the bottom, and they were *so proud* of their selection when we got home.

They loved that goldfish like crazy. They'd talk to it every time they had the chance. First thing in the morning, they had to go and check on their goldfish friend. Before bed, they had to tell him goodnight, as kids do. They were completely smitten with the little thing, and they made that very clear.

Well, that first fish didn't live very long at all. They say those fish are supposed to live for years, but this one barely lasted in our home. Maybe my tank was the wrong size, or the water wasn't right, or maybe the fish was just unhealthy, perhaps it needed a supply of oxygen—we'll never know. The first time had to be a fluke, so we got a second goldfish to keep the kids happy. After all, I had seen just how much they cared for their little buddy, and who was I to deny them that pleasure of enjoying the company of a pet in their lives?

Well, that one didn't last very long either. I don't know what we did wrong, but it was clear to me after the second goldfish that we weren't cut out to be goldfish owners, and fine by me. It was no skin off my back—I didn't really want a pet in the first place. I knew it'd be a hassle, but I was really just in it for the kids, to give them something that they wanted to make them happy.

Of course, the kids weren't happy with that answer. They pouted, and they sighed dramatically as kids tend to do, and they begged for a pet. When were they asked what they wanted for their birthdays? They want another pet. They'd do everything that they could to let us know that all they wanted was an animal friend to call their own. Didn't I know that all of their friends had pets? And everyone on TV had pets, so they needed one too?

Eventually, I gave in again. We got a cute little bird this time. The bird was bound to be more resilient, wasn't it? I figured it would somehow live longer than the fish, and it was nice to look at, too. So, off to the pet store we went again. We picked out everything that we would need for our pet bird, and the kids picked out the bird that they wanted.

He was a pretty little thing, and Salam was his name. He was friendly enough, and the kids were just as smitten with him as with the fish. I'd hear them telling me all about what Salam did that day when I'd get home from work, and admittedly, it was quite adorable. I liked the bird, and after it survived the first few weeks, longer than the fish ever did, I started to relax.

Unfortunately, that poor little bird was not meant for the weather of California. He was meant to live somewhere warm and humid, and the winter weather was not kind to him. He had been looking somewhat sickly for a while that winter, but one day I realized that he wasn't doing well. He was slow, breathing heavily, and lethargic. He didn't want to eat, and he didn't really respond much to being a pet.

I started to worry. We couldn't have another pet die—not like that. So, I took him with me in the car. I tried to make him comfortable as I went from vet to vet, looking for someone, anyone, who would be willing to treat our little birdy friend.

I was dreading the conversations that I was afraid would come next. One moment I'd tell myself that poor little Salam wouldn't die, and the next, I was steeling myself for the inevitable. I did my best to figure out how to balance expectations with what was happening.

Suffering animals are a bit of a sore point for me. I hate seeing them suffering and dying, and being there next to poor little Salam as I desperately tried to find someone who left a mark on me. I still remember the moment when he seemed to be getting worse. He was breathing and moving slowly, and then he just closed his eyes, and he was gone.

Death is difficult for anyone, and I found myself distraught over the poor little bird's death. I questioned whether I had done everything that I could or if things could have been different. Of course, that kind of dwelling never helps anyone, and I had to push it out of my mind as well. I needed to cope, to be strong for my kids, but my mental health made that much harder than I could have expected.

For the next several weeks, I was anxious and depressed. I reflected upon death as a whole. I knew that I would also eventually die. Would it be soon? Would it be as sudden as poor fish and Salam? Would I have any warning? Would it be preventable? Of course, the more that I dwelled on the idea of death, the more that panic seemed to find me. I'd have full-blown panic attacks over the idea, and that, of course, left my sense of stability that much more rocked and that much more off kilter. I couldn't believe it—another pet had died on our watch. Maybe we just shouldn't try anymore. Of course, my children weren't very happy about that idea. About a month after poor Salam had passed in my car, my children were on to their next scheme. They had presented me with their newest grand idea: A cat.

Yes, a cat! Their answer to their bird and their fish dying was to try getting a cat instead! I told them no. No way were we bringing a cat into our home. A cat was a big responsibility, didn't they know? It's not as easy as just giving a fish a few flakes of food or keeping a birdcage clean. There was so much more to it than just that. Cats needed real good care; they needed to be bathed and brushed and have their nails trimmed. They needed a clean litter box, plenty of space to play, and it would mean a lot of cat fur to vacuum! I told them that there was no way we were bringing all of that responsibility into our home unnecessarily and that there was no way that they could convince me to do so.

Was it really about the work? Maybe a little bit, truthfully, but the biggest problem that I had with getting a cat was that I didn't want to see another animal die. We had already done those three times in a row, and what if it happened again? What if one of the kids left the door open and the cat got out and was hit by a car? What if *I* were the one who hit him with my car when I was coming or leaving? What if he chewed up a wire and was electrocuted? What if someone sat on him, or if he ate something that he shouldn't have? What if he was just sickly and died due to natural causes?

The idea of bringing that kind of uncertainty into my home again was something I couldn't bear, and all of the intrusive thoughts were there to remind me that the last thing that I needed to be doing was bringing another living thing into our home may also die.

But you've never met my kids. They're very persuasive, you see, and before long, the pressure was too much to bear. Sure, I was terrified of seeing a cat die in my home, but I was also dealing with the pressure of three young kids who just wanted to have their own friend to play with at home. I had to choose between coping with my own struggles and my own mental health by avoidance or choosing to face my fear head-on and make that sacrifice so that my children could have what they wanted, and their pressured persuasions won out.

After a lot of deliberation and talking back and forth, they finally wore me down and convinced me that yes, we could get a cat, and we went to select one. Of all the cats that we saw, and of all the options, the one that caught the attention of my family was a gorgeous long-haired cat. His black and white fur was luxuriously long, and he purred when his head was scratched just the right way.

That day, we brought home our newest family member, whom we named Felfel. Felfel is our greatest new sweetheart. While I tried my hardest to keep my distance, not wanting to let myself get caught up in getting attached to another pet that I was convinced might also die and leave another gap in my heart, I couldn't help but adore it. Loving him came naturally. He seemed to sense that I needed something more in my life. It was as if he knew that I had this empty space in my heart that needed to be filled with something warm and full of love, and there he was.

Next to my family, the cat became my best bud at home. When everyone's gone, he's quick to be by my side, and he seeks me out whenever I'm not around. He chooses to play with me, and he sleeps next to me at night. Though I was hesitant to admit it, he won me over. He made me realize that sometimes, even if things do die eventually, it is worth opening up our hearts. Yes, we will hurt when we lose them, but the resulting love that you get in the meantime is worth it.

I found myself happier with Felfel around, and he integrated seamlessly into our family. I suddenly found myself with a new friend, and with how often he follows me around, he's almost like a new chaperone—someone there to supervise me when I need it. It's almost like he can sense when I need him the most, and there he is with his fluffy fur and his deep, soothing purrs when I need someone in the moment. He became our newest family member, and he is irreplaceable.

Chapter 5: Can You Say That Again?

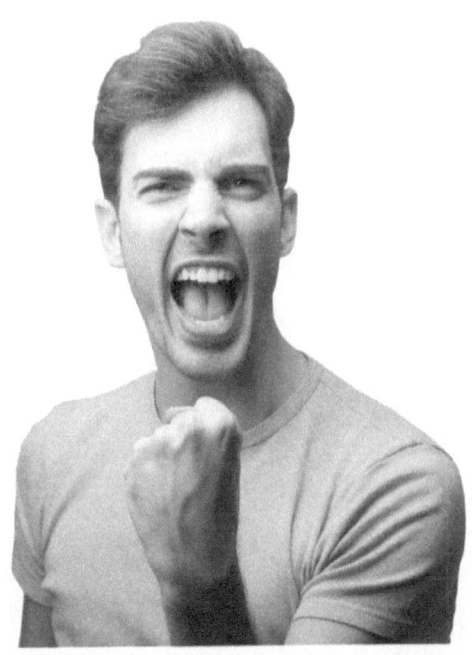

Religion is one of those topics that a lot of people kind of skirt around. After all, there are so many different beliefs and perceptions of the interpretations that surround them. It is a tough topic to talk about with people who may not agree with you. It is one of those subjects that people will vehemently oppose if you bring it up the wrong way. Have you ever seen how upset people can get if you reference religion to someone who isn't personally religious, or if you try to skirt around it to a devout believer?

Even if it is a tough topic to bridge, I personally am so much of a devout believer that I cannot live without God. A world where there is no God is one in which I wouldn't know how to navigate. How do you go on when there isn't a purpose? What do you do when you feel like your life is meaningless or like you have no real reason to exist? God gives me that meaning and purpose. I know that I have a purpose, even when I may not know what it may be, because God made me for a reason.

Now, don't get me wrong—I sympathize with the agnostics and the atheists. They might manage to free themselves at a particular time, but at what cost? To free oneself from the rule of God is to fall from grace, as is said. It is to claim that you are purposeless, random, and utterly alone. The atheist doesn't have someone to talk to when they are sitting alone, with no one there besides themselves. They don't get the comfort of knowing that there is someone greater than themselves who cares about them. It is a simpler way of life. They may not have to worry about what God thinks or how they live their lives, but that simplicity comes at a cost. When all goes wrong, they have no one to ask for help. They have no one there to help them discover what comes next.

I believe that God is there for us, even when everyone else abandons us. Even in our darkest moments, when we are contemplating things that we'd never want to speak out loud, God is there, listening, and waiting patiently. When our family is gone, and our friends are nowhere to be found, I can rest well, knowing that I have God there by my side, supporting me and pushing me forward.

I've tried to talk about this with my friends. I went to my religious buddies to have talks about death, but they were less than helpful. I wanted to discuss my fear of the unknown and the fear of death, but they were quick to tell me that as a believer in God, I should know that it is all in His plan and that He will not allow me to die until it is my time. Why wouldn't I be willing to think that way, they'd ask me? Why am I so quick to talk about being afraid? Didn't I know that by being afraid of death, I was questioning God's judgment? I had to believe that His plan would be right for me, and that was that.

Well, I didn't think it was so open and shut at the time. Yes, I knew that I needed to trust in God and that God would never let me down. But that didn't make dying any less scary! Yes, there is an afterlife, but what about my life here and now? What about my children, my wife, and Felfel? What would happen to them when I was gone? I could accept that God had a plan for everything and for us all, while I was still concerned about the aftermath. Even if it were all according to His plan, that didn't mean that my death wouldn't happen and that my death wouldn't hurt people who love me the most. Every day, every hour, every breath brings me closer to death, and I know that to be the case. But, at that time, I couldn't live with that fact. The idea that I would die one day was paralyzing to me, but I know now that my friends were right. I know now that the answer about my death isn't as scary as I made it out to be.

Even though I always thought that my friends were wrong in implying that I was overcomplicating things, I knew that their advice was not enough to help me. Their words alone did not make me feel any better, no more secure, or any more capable of feeling relief than anything else. I knew that they all meant well, but they didn't help my situation. I still questioned death. I still feared it. I dwelled on it, and it controlled my life. I felt like every moment of every day was tiptoeing around these problems in hopes of figuring out what I could do to prevent my untimely death. I was afraid of it, and that fear ultimately ruled my life in ways that it should not have allowed it to do. Of course, thoughts have a great way of controlling themselves and spiraling out of control, and that is exactly what happened to me. I was unable to prevent it, and I had no sense of control over what I was doing. There was no way for me to be able to manage myself. No matter how hard I tried, I couldn't make myself feel any better.

God had a different plan for me than allowing me to remain lost in thought and ruminating over my eventual demise. He, as He always does, had a plan to help me get through those darkest moments, and that time His plan was to teach me a very important lesson, and I learned that lesson through my psychiatrist. We all know that God works in strange and mysterious ways, but now that I'm on the other side of the journey, I can see what He was doing. I can see that he brought me to that appointment, to that one doctor, for a very good reason, and that reason was incredibly compelling for me. That reason became my lifesaver. And so, off I went to my doctor's visit that changed my life and the course of my experience with depression.

One day, I visited him for a routine appointment to get my medication refilled and ensure that it was working correctly. I went to the appointment with my thoughts weighing heavily on me. I was terrified! Death would be coming eventually, and I knew it—I'd never know when it would be, but it would ultimately and inevitably happen. At the time, I couldn't live with that fact. I just could not accept that truth. I went through the appointment like normal, and I was caught off guard when I was asked: "How are you feeling nowadays, Magdy?"

I was surprised, and I hesitated. I took a moment to gather my thoughts and then answered him with exactly what was weighing so heavily on me: "I'm feeling like I will die at any moment." I meant it, too. My anxiety had me thoroughly convinced that it would happen soon. I was terrified just getting through my day-to-day life, and I had no idea how to navigate through such intense feelings. I had no idea what I could possibly do to help myself. Normally, I would have lied, I would have shrugged with a feigned smile and said that I was doing alright, but this time I felt compelled to tell him the truth.

The words flowed from my mouth before I was able to stop them, and after I finished speaking, I waited with bated breath, convinced that he'd have a resolution for my problem when I replied. Was it wrong to talk to the doctor in such a manner? Was it wrong to tell him what I was really thinking and feeling? Maybe, but God had it right that time. I believe that God was there with me when I had spoken, or how else could I have said exactly the right thing at the right time to get exactly the answer that I didn't know that I needed?

He didn't seem fazed by my answer at all. His response was easy, in fact, too easy for someone who was just told that his patient was concerned about dying. He looked at me briefly and replied, "I don't see you dying anytime soon. You are in fantastic physical shape, and you will live a long life. You're healthy." With that simple reassurance, he turned back to his computer and started typing away.

I left with those words hanging over my head. They were there, filling me with confusion and doubt. I doubted myself, and I doubted his words at the same time. My anxiety had me convinced that death was inevitable, that it would happen at any time, and that I would never be able to prevent it. My anxiety convinced me that death was imminent, that every time I had a panic attack, it could be the end of me, and that I had a precious few days left.

At the same time, I had to grapple with what my doctor had told me. How could he know? I had to wonder about it. How could he have been able to say that with such certainty? I could have been hit by a car in the parking lot as soon as I left the office! There were so many variables, and why would I have felt like I was going to die every time I had a panic attack if I weren't actually dying? How could I possibly believe that what this doctor had to say was true?

But the truth is that he was correct. The more I grappled with what he had to say, and the more that I pondered his words and figured out what he meant, the more reassured I felt. I thought back to one of the several times when I ended up in the hospital during a panic attack. I was terrified. My heart was pounding. My chest felt tight, and I felt like I couldn't breathe. I had been convinced at the time that my heart was failing, and I went to the hospital.

They had referred me to a cardiologist. I'm not sure if they thought there was something wrong with my heart, or if they were just covering their bases, but they wanted to check me out. I went along, desperate for the answers that would tell me what was wrong with me. I went with hopes of discovering if there was actually something that I could have done about my physical health, or if there were any answers as to what was going on with me.

I remember when I went there. I was sitting after all the tests and waiting for the results. I was convinced that they would tell me my heart was failing or that I had had a heart attack or something else more horrible, but the truth was that I was overthinking it. I still remember my doctor coming in to give me the good news. He told me that my heart was perfectly healthy, but he didn't have much else to say about it.

I also remember wondering what would come next. I still believed that even if I wasn't having a heart attack right then, I would have one soon. I knew that death was imminent, and even getting the A-Okay from the cardiologist was not enough to assuage that fear and doubt. That didn't do anything at all to help me feel better. All it did was make me feel more like I would be dead before I knew it, and it made me feel more as if my death would be even more unpredictable. At least if he had told me that my heart was in poor health, I would have been able to prepare! Despite the good news,

I remember leaving the cardiologist's office with that same pit of dread in my gut without any sense of feeling better.

That appointment with the cardiologist came back to me as I walked out of the psychiatrist's office, and I realized something. Now I had had two doctors tell me that, in terms of my physical condition, I was perfectly healthy. They had both assured me that there was nothing to worry about, and at that moment, I had an epiphany. How could I possibly die in the near future if both of my doctors had told me that I was healthy?

As I walked out of the office that day, I realized that my psychiatrist, who had been trying for ages to get the medication that I was on just right to treat my anxiety and depression, had suddenly flipped the switch in my mind. He probably didn't realize it at the time, but he was a turning point for my mindset in my journey against the anxiety and depression that I faced. I knew from him that I would die eventually, but not now. Not soon. Not even in the near future. He made it clear to me that I had plenty of time in my life to survive, to live, and to enjoy my life with my loved ones.

The funny thing is, my doctor, my not-so-religious psychiatrist, helped me more than my religious friends ever did in clearing that one question from my conscience. I found that I could finally rest easy knowing that I would be just fine in the long run. I knew that I would be able to relax a bit, and I'd be able to accept the truth about my life. It was like all of that weight that I had been carrying on my shoulders was finally released, and resultantly I found that I was able to do so much more with my life. By letting go of that anxiety and that pain that had followed me around, I could do so much more. I was able to finally breathe again. I could finally get back to living.

My first question was answered by my second lifesaver—my psychiatrist. I knew that I would not die soon.

Chapter 6: Pushing Up to the Surface

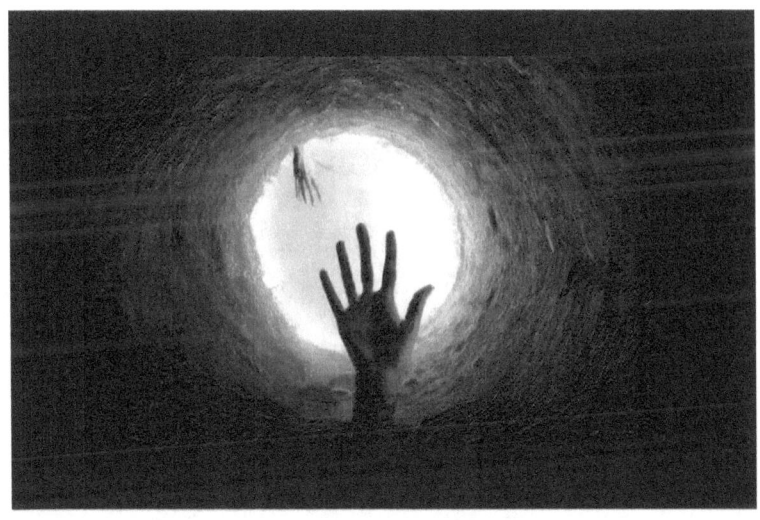

My dear friend, the psychologist, was a very systematic man. He was the kind of person who would document every moment of what he was doing, and he would monitor his progress. He would also write down when he did something and how it worked for him. He loved the structure of schedules and regularly followed them on his own. He would work to ensure that he was following up, no matter what the cost. Rain or shine, if he said that he was doing something, he would do it like clockwork. He is a brilliant man. Rigid and strict, but smart and compassionate as well. He would have to be a good psychologist, and considering the impact he had on my life as my final lifesaver, he was a fantastic one as well.

When I first talked to my dear friend, he had two requirements for me. After I told him about my symptoms, he reminded me of two key things that I needed to do every day. No matter what happened, I had to spend half an hour walking, even if it was pouring rain, and I would also have to write in my journal every day. I thought his advice was somewhat silly, but I agreed to do it. He demanded it, so I did it. After all, he was the expert, right?

His instructions for me to journal were simple: I had to sit down every day and write. It didn't matter what it was that I was to write; he didn't want me to merely think about it or what it was that I transcribed. All he wanted me to do was write, write, and write. I did that a lot, and every day without fail. I will write about what I did and even what I ate. I'd go over how I was working with myself and how I could do better. I'd write down my feelings, actions, and just about anything else that could have possibly been beneficial to me, and yet I still didn't feel like it would help. After all, writing about that silly thing my kids did, or what I ate for dinner, didn't provide much insight into what was happening with me as far as I could tell. Still, my friend had asked me to do so, and so I did. Every day, like clockwork, I took my walk, and then I wrote down everything about what I did each day. I also wrote in the evenings, but I didn't notice anything changing about myself. I didn't feel better. I didn't feel any different at all.

When my psychiatrist friend came to visit me, I was excited, but also a bit nervous. My journal wasn't helping at all, and I had to figure out how to tell him. He flew to visit me from Arizona, and he sat down to review my written journal. He would quietly go over what I had written, reading over all of the entries, and then discuss what may have caused my anxiety attack that day. It seemed like he was convinced that my anxiety could have been triggered by just about anything, and some of the things that he said seemed so off the wall, I couldn't believe them.

Maybe my anxiety is because of television, so he suggested after reading about I watch the news for a while before my panic attacks. I can't remember what had been on the news that day, but he seemed to think that the bad news could have been the cause. Perhaps, but who knows? I wasn't convinced.

Maybe my anxiety was due to the spicy food I had for dinner, as he suggested after another reading of that entry. He told me to eliminate spicy foods from my diet as well because that could have been the cause. The more he read from my journal, the more he seemed to restrict me. He told me to stop watching the news and to eat more spicy foods. He wanted to know if they were, or were not, influencing me. He went by the book, as is said, for after all, he was a psychologist, and he wanted the best for me. Even when I thought his suggestions were strange, I listened to him because he seemed to know what was in my best interest at heart.

He was ultimately my third lifesaver on this journey, and he worked with me tirelessly. He never gave up on me or my anxiety issues, constantly looking for the cause so that I could feel and be better, and looking back upon it, I had to be grateful for his efforts. He was so deliberate about everything, and he had neither a reason nor an obligation to travel to visit from Arizona. Yet, there he was at my side, especially when I needed him the most. He was always there for me. I was attentive to what he had to say, and I worked to ensure that I would get better. Slowly but surely, I did improve, but it took time and patience.

One summer afternoon, my anxiety hit hard. I felt like I couldn't breathe. I was convinced I was dying. I wasn't sure what had set me off, but one thing was for certain: I was not stable. Usually, when my anxiety was bad like that, my wife and I had a plan. I'd usually drive myself to the hospital because my wife had our children to look after. If I couldn't drive or I didn't feel safe driving, I could contact my cousin (M.I.), who lived directly next door to me. However, that afternoon he wasn't home yet, so I had to wait for him for thirty agonizing minutes. I waited until he arrived home from work, and as soon as I knew he was back, I called him.

He was there for me immediately. He didn't even change out of his work clothes. He asked me to he would wait for me outside my house, and when I got into his car, he drove directly to the ER. By then, I was a familiar face at ER, but they still had to do their due diligence of getting me admitted. They couldn't treat me without first making certain that my symptoms weren't caused by something that would have been a bit more pressing. I had to go over the symptoms again and wait for them to perform my routine checkup.

I told them that I was there for my chest pain. They took my vitals, and my blood pressure was ideal, and I was told that I didn't appear to be suffering from a heart attack. Because they didn't deem me to be an urgent admittance, I was required to wait. They put a little plastic ID bracelet on my wrist and sent me to the waiting room.

Two hours later, I was still sitting there, stressed and confused. I looked to my cousin with frustration and remembered asking him: "Is this how they treat a person with a possible or real heart attack?" I was sarcastic, but it was definitely what I was feeling. I was ultimately dismissed from the hospital with the usual advice. They told me that if I was concerned, then I should contact my doctor or care provider to get stress or anxiety medication, and that was that. No help, no answers, nothing.

So, I left feeling frustrated and hopeless, having to leave unattended. I was sent back home without much else to go with, and I would be lying if I said that I was surprised. It seemed like the medical world thought of my anxiety and depression as nothing but a mere inconvenience to me, and while my family, closest to me, was incredibly supportive, I sometimes struggled with outsiders.

That night, I got to meet with my friend (S.D.). He had sent me a concerned message earlier that day that he had heard I was in the ER and was worried about what had happened to me. I told him my story and what had occurred. I told him that I had been suffering from anxiety and depression again and that I was so concerned about what was going on within myself. He seemed surprised to hear that about me and asked to see me that night.

"Of course," I replied! I would always make time for my friends. So, that night he arrived around 10:00 that evening, which was rather late, but it was nice to catch up with him. He was with me for six hours and didn't leave until 4 am. We spent the entire night just chatting with each other. We talked about all sorts of things, but the primary purpose was to talk to me about his story, essentially what he had gone through.

He told me about his own story and surprised me by telling me that he, too, was diagnosed with anxiety and depression. At first, I was just tired and wanted him to hurry through it until I realized that he was telling me a story that sounded incredibly similar to my own. He told me of his treatments, of the triggers for his own anxiety attacks, and more. He had suffered just as much as I had, and I was in shock.

My friend had always seemed so strong! I had never known that he was suffering. I had never even thought that someone like him would have struggled with anxiety and depression, and yet, here we were! We were sitting and talking about what he had needed to do and how he did it. He also told me about his lowest lows, and I realized that he and I were verily more alike than I had initially thought. We had always been good friends, but at that moment, I realized that we shared something in common, a bond that not everyone has. I had a friend who knew exactly what I was feeling and how I was suffering. I had a friend who was able to understand what I was going through and how I could influence myself to be a better person. He was there, living proof that life could be better.

I watched him in awe for a while. After six hours of storytelling and listening, at four in the morning when I was ready to sleep, I found myself staring at him, wondering if he knew just how much of what he had said to me had resonated. I presumed that he must have known on some level and that he more clearly understood me. He both went through what I went through. He got treatment. He got better. He got better and became so well that I hadn't even known there had been something wrong with him in the first place! That was amazing to me. It was a surprise that I was able to know that about him. I considered how he had behaved and realized the truth was that he was able to do so much more because he was able to treat himself. He had gotten through to the end of his story and arrived at the other side of his situation. How?

I realized that I needed to know that information. I needed to know his secret. I needed to know how he was doing now and if it was possible that there was light at the end of this tunnel for me. If he could defeat his own depression, could I do the same? Was it possible that I could actually achieve a sense of normalcy again? It seemed like an impossibility for so long, and yet here he was, sitting with me as normal as he could be. He seemed so confident, so comfortable, and so *normal*. I knew I needed to be like him. I needed to know his secret.

But what if he's just pretending? This thought hit me like a ton of bricks. Is it possible that things weren't as normal as he was saying? Is it possible that even though he looked normal on the outside, he was really just as frustrated, just as upset, and just as anxious as ever on the inside? I doubted that success in treating anxiety was so achievable. I wanted to believe it was possible, but at the same time, how could it be? It had always managed to hold me down more than anything else. It was almost crippling with how bad it got at times. How could he possibly be in a position where it was so easy to let it go?

Ultimately, I realized that the only way I'd know was if I asked. And so, at the end of his story, I looked at him for a moment. The silence hung in the air as we looked at each other. Then, I finally asked the question that had been lingering on my mind for so long: "How are you doing now?"

I realized that I was afraid to hear the answer. As soon as the words came out of my mouth, I realized that the answer could make or break me. Would I be able to accept it if things weren't actually alright? Would I be able to move on if he told me that he was still being dragged down with the same crisis? Would I be alright if he told me that I would never be able to get back to normal? The impending answer was terrifying, and at that moment, I was both hopeful and doubtful. I held my breath, waiting to hear what he had to say. "I'm fine. I'm back to normal."

And just like that, with those two sentences, the weight that had been dragging me down for so long was gone. Just like that, relief crashed over me so heavily that I was able to believe that everything would be fine if I kept moving forward. I would be just fine—I just had to be willing to accept my situation and keep looking toward the future. I had living proof, right there in front of me, that normalcy could be achieved.

"My God", I remember thinking to myself as I stared at him in shock, I can be normal just like him. It was so relieving to hear that I would eventually be just fine. It was as if so much weight had been taken off my chest with the realization that I will be able to eventually be better in my own time. All I had to do was work for it, and I could achieve it.

I don't think my friend realized the gravity of what he had told me and how I had taken it. I don't think he realized at the moment that he genuinely saved my life with his own journey. His story was literally life-changing for me— hearing that he had successfully come out of his agony, I knew that it was possible for me as well. I knew that I wasn't going to be stuck like this forever and that normalcy was there waiting for me. I could see the light shining just by seeing him in front of me, and I could see that my life was worth living and that, like him, I would also be alright.

I had already learned that I wasn't dying any time soon, thanks to my psychiatrist. Now, hearing what he had to say, I realized that normalcy was possible for me as well. That brought closure that I hadn't realized I could achieve. That gave me a sense that I'll be able to do better, be better, feel better, and live better than I had realized. I also knew that I could be back to normal—I could be a crisis-free spouse, parent, and the person that I yearned to be, all by having heard what my psychiatrist friend had told me.

As I continued to look at him, I realized that I could feel the ease that I had been missing for so long. Life will be bright and colorful again. I could see that the world was unfolding in front of me, surrounding me with hope. I could see that there was a purpose in continuing to persevere to achieve full recovery.

He inspired me to keep on fighting for myself. It wasn't always easy, but when I struggled the most, I knew that I could think of SD and realize that I was on the right track. Even when I felt like the world was crashing down around me, I would be able to think to myself: "Well, what would SD have done?" Or I would think about what he had actually done to get himself out of the rut that he was in. It didn't take me long to discover the truth, and I was able to use it to my advantage.

My questions and concerns were answered. My journey no longer felt as bleak as it had been before. I no longer felt like I was doomed to suffer or that I'd be stuck, held back, or unable to succeed. All I had to do was ensure that I was working toward the recovery that I wanted to achieve, and as soon as I could do that, I would be just fine.

Part II Closure

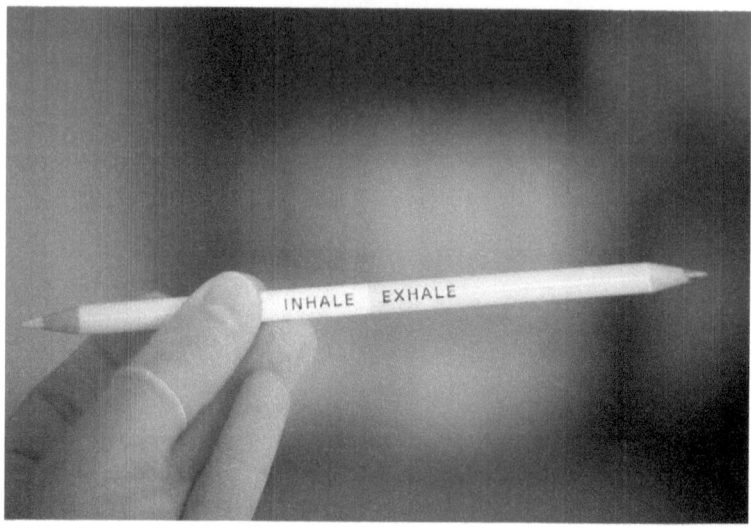

And that brings me to the end of Part II of my journey with depression and anxiety. As you can see, depression and anxiety are not easy. They can be terrifying. They can be soul-crushing. They can be terrifying. You can wind up feeling like you are about to die. You can end up feeling like there is no way to continue living. You can end up feeling like you are the worst possible person in the world with no possible way to succeed in life, and when you are in that position, you can get quite desperate.

I know that desperation very well, and I know that there is nothing like it. I also know now that the desperation that lies behind your anxiety and depression is nothing but a lie. It is there, whispering to you, to lie to you? It doesn't want to help you. It doesn't want you to be happy. What it doesn't tell you, however, is that you can achieve happiness. You can achieve that inner peace that you once enjoyed. I did it, and you can, too.

My journey was very long. It was full of lows that I thought I'd never be able to surmount. I was weighed down by those two questions that I couldn't wrap my mind around or grapple with. I was stuck underneath the crushing pressure of being unable to do and be better. I couldn't behave better. I couldn't be better. I couldn't get past the present moment of dread, of panic, and of hopelessness.

I used to wonder if I would die soon. I didn't know then, but now I do know that I would not be dying any time soon. I know now that I'm healthy, that I'm able to do what I need to do. I know that I'm able to be the "me" that I need to be and that I'm able to do so with ease. All I needed to do was hear from my doctor that I would be just fine.

Would I be able to get back to normal? I doubted it in the beginning, but I know now that the doubt that I felt was nothing but my own fears weighing on me. I know now that the doubt that I felt was not due to anxiety and depression that were trying to keep me in that pit. Normalcy is there and attainable. Normalcy can be found—you just have to learn what you have to do to search for and achieve it, and as soon as you do that, you will know that you can do so much better.

Now, I've shared my story with you. I've walked you through what my own thought processes were. The thoughts that I had were difficult to cope with at times. They were tough to really analyze and figure out. However, in learning to work through my thoughts, I discovered how I could grapple with my own feelings, my own insecurities, and my own fears. Through the influence and help of my devoted wife, my dear cat Felfel, my psychiatrist R.D., my psychologist K.S., and my great friend, S.D., my life was saved. My life was something that I was able to take control of once more, and I was able to pull it from the grasp of my depression and anxiety.

You now know how I was able to get through everything that held me down. You've read how I was able to begin to better myself. You learned what it took for me to reach that point of knowing that I could succeed and get back to a normal life.

If you're reading this book because you are currently suffering on your own, then hopefully you can begin to find some solace in knowing that all hope is not lost. Hopefully, at this point, you can see that your journey is only just beginning. Your life isn't over because you have depression or anxiety—it is only beginning. Your life isn't going to be destroyed because of your feelings—it will just begin to work for you. If you want to be able to be the best person that you can be, all you have to do is begin to work on improving yourself.

Hopefully, too, you will now no longer feel as alone as you once did. You no longer feel like you have to just barely make your way through life. You can see that comfort is possible and attainable if you know what you are doing. You can do better! You can live again! Freedom, happiness, and closure are possible to achieve. You just have to be determined to keep fighting, and you have to keep working at it. Never forget that you have this power and ability. Never forget that your life has meaning and value and that you have ways of beginning to improve yourself!

Thank you for taking the time to read through my story. It was difficult to get it all out there for scrutinizing, but I have chosen to share it because I believe that there is very real value in doing so. I believe that there is very real value in being able to talk about what I went through in hopes of making other people feel more like they are capable of achieving their own successes. My one hope is to ensure that other people feel that they are able to fight throughout this journey on their own, without shame and without feeling like they are weak. At this point in my journey, as you have read, it's all about time. It's all about me walking toward the brighter side, and you can join me on that journey. You can cross that line to achieve the same success, where life has color and meaning again as it did for me.

Part III "Climbing the Mountain"

Part II Recap

At last, we reach the end of my story, but before we go over that, let's take a look at where my journey has gone thus far. My story started with me on the brink of destruction. Depression and anxiety are two beasts that I'd never want to wish on even my worst enemy. They held us down. They whisper in our ears, telling us all of the lies that they can to keep us back and make us believe that we really are nothing but dead weight, that our families would be better without us, or that we'll never be happy or able to love our lives.

In the first part of my journey, I came to terms with my feelings of anxiety and depression. I recognized that I had a problem and that there was hope for me to get better. I started to realize that what I was going through was more common than I thought, that there were people out there who could help me, and that there were ways that I could start to recover. It all started one day on an airplane flight. It was a normal day for me because I traveled often. But, it took just one day—no, just minutes—to seemingly change my life forever. The small airplane was in severe turbulence, and it was so horrible that I was terrified that I would die. I wasn't the only one, either. There were grown men crying. Everyone was silent on the airplane, and though we all walked off that aircraft, I know now that a part of me figuratively died on it. I became anxious and depressed. I had panic attacks. I had to give up on much of what I did before. Traveling for business? No way! I could no longer do it. The mere thought of flying was enough to induce panic. Part I was like my death. It was my sinking into depression and being wholly consumed by it. I was unable to be the person that I wanted to be, and I felt totally defeated.

In Part II of my journey, I grappled with two questions that I couldn't get out of my mind. I was stuck wondering how soon I would die, and if it wasn't to be soon, then was it possible to live a normal life again? These questions were difficult to deal with. It was hard to address them, to feel like I could be the person that I once was before, but I had no choice. I have a family that needs me, and though the depression and anxiety might deceive me about them, I know that they are there and in need of my presence.

As I worked through the next part of my journey, I was stuck in my mind as I ruminated over those two simple questions. I'd have panic attacks. I'd break down. I'd feel like I was dying. Ultimately, I had three people who changed my life during that time of my ordeal. They were able to help me not only to see the light, to find that hope when I felt like it was gone forever, but also to help me to finally acknowledge the truth about my situation.

It all began with my dear sweet wife. She was my rock throughout everything. She took our wedding vows of "…in sickness and in health…" in stride, and she was always there for me when I needed her. She was there to console me and calmly talk me through my panic attacks, and she was there to remind and assure me that I was not alone. When she wasn't enough to help me get past a panic attack, she was there to help me get to the hospital to be stabilized. She helped me more than she'll ever know, and I shall be eternally thankful for her unyielding support.

My psychiatrist, R.D., also helped save my life, not physically, but mentally. He answered my first question that I was stuck on with ease. He was so nonchalant about it, never missing a beat when I told him that I felt like my own death was imminent. He reminded me that my charts indicated that I was healthy, that I looked fine, and that he would be very surprised if I died in the near future due to a body failure. However, had he only said that in passing, he was nonetheless able to help me. I was able to answer that first question: Would I die soon? No! He taught me that I'd be just fine and that my body was in perfect shape for a **long and** happy life.

My psychologist friend helped me immensely as well. He helped me figure out a schedule, regimens, and routines to try to combat my anxiety. He took me seriously, even when I was afraid that no one would. He reminded me that I would eventually be just fine, that I would also be able to defeat my problems, and he pushed me to be healthier, to take action, and to live my life to the fullest extent possible. Without him, I'm not certain I would have managed to get as far as I did. To him, too, I am also eternally thankful. He was a lifesaver for me.

Finally, we arrived at my dear friend, SD. He not only saved my life, but he also gave me hope. He helped me to see the door that I needed to pass through. He taught me that there is happiness and normalcy after overcoming anxiety and depression. He showed me that I could get back to normal, that I could find a way to achieve living my life without constant fear or anxiety, and all I needed to do was work through it with patience and determination. He was another lifesaver who shared his own story with me, and he assured me that I would be just fine.

That brings us to Part III: Climbing the Mountain. What a mountain my journey was! Through my pain, suffering, trauma, confusion, and desperation, I realized there was one spot that kept me returning my attention to - "The Door." That door I'd see in my mind was the doorway that would take me out of my own depression. All I needed to do was reach out and open it. It was still too far away to reach, but I knew that over time, I would get there.

Through experience, I learned that taking baby steps should never be underestimated. Yes, they might seem so small and insignificant, but if you put enough of those baby steps together, you can begin to see big progress. Think about this book for a moment, this book is comprised of chapters. Those chapters consist of paragraphs, and they contain sentences. Those sentences are a compilation of words. And those words are made up of letters. Baby steps are like individual letters that must be put together to create the whole journey. Little things come together to create the whole collective.

Now, there were a few setbacks. Progress ebbs and flows, and sometimes, I felt like I had completely regressed entirely with no real way to fix the problem, but the truth is, the little things, those baby steps, help you to recover. They put you back on track. The final stage in my journey was a remarkable time that tested my willingness, determination, and my deepest desire to move toward total recovery. It was dependent upon the environment that I was in, and while I may not be able to change the world around me, I can change where I am in the world. I could walk away from anxiety and depression. I could choose to open that healing door. I could be free from that constricted life. All I had to do was be strong enough to take control of my situation, to manage my anxiety and depression, and when I did that, I realized that I could get far ahead.

Chapter 7: Create My Cozy World

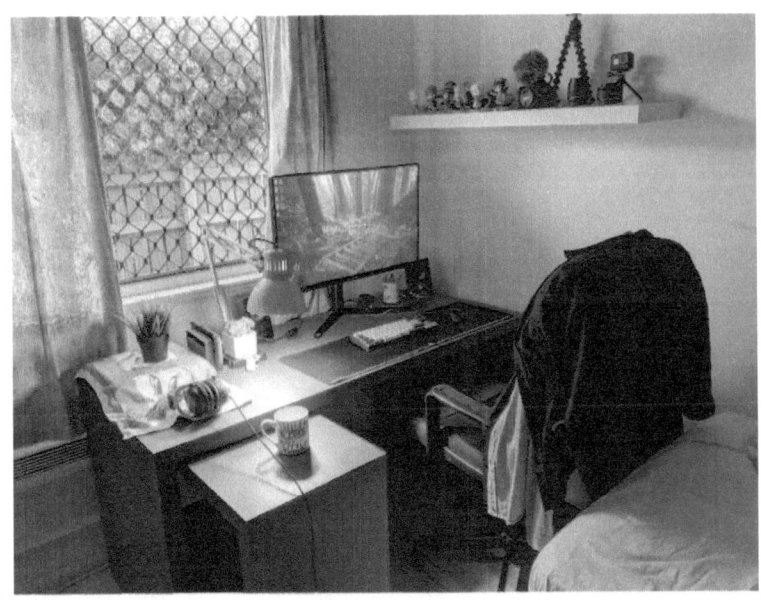

Anxiety and depression can leave your mind in an incredible and inhospitable place. The thoughts of negativity, of thinking the worst of every situation, weigh heavily on the mind, and they can drag any semblance of happiness that you may have found right back into the pits of deeper depression. I wanted to spend time with other people, but at the same time, I could hear that voice in the back of my mind telling me not to bother, that it was a waste of my time, and that I wasn't wanted anyway.

We're a social species. We crave having a connection with other people, and even in my anxiety, I craved it. I was desperate to get that attention and connection, and yet, I found it so difficult to achieve. I knew I needed to do so, but it was scary. Sure, my visits to the ER had been steadily decreasing, but I felt like my anxiety attacks got stronger. I felt like even though I knew I wasn't dying, I still felt just as scared, just as miserable, and just as ready for the other proverbial shoe to fall. It was like my body was trying desperately to clear itself of a toxin to be free once and for all. I had to get worse before I got better, but if I was able to survive through it, there would be better days ahead. SD had told me that—he had told me that normalcy was there on the sidelines and that I would be able to achieve it again if I tried. He told me that I would be able to become that normal person again, and I had to believe him.

Of course, anyone who knows the feeling of depression knows that it's hard to get past it. It's next to impossible to reason with yourself when you have anxiety and depression convincing you that you aren't worth it or whispering that it's not worth even bothering because everyone only pities you instead. It's so hard to tow that line between being afraid of socializing or wanting to be left in your own sorrows, but still looking for some way that you can connect to others. It is a crucial time—you have to figure out how best to meet wants and needs while still trying to juggle your mental health, and it is not easy by any means.

The Little Habits

In the early days, after my diagnosis, my wife didn't want to leave me alone. It felt like she was always making excuses to stick around so she would be present if I needed her. To be brutally honest, I wasn't really comfortable enough to be alone anyway, and she did not want to leave; it only meant that I didn't have to voice those words out loud. I didn't have to tell her that I was afraid that I wanted her nearby, because she didn't want to be away either. I wasn't comfortable sitting at home, all alone, waiting for another false heart attack to end my life. I wanted to at least have someone around who could drive me to the hospital or call 911 if it was truly urgent.

But that kind of stagnancy, that requirement of a grown adult to be supervised by others, was not healthy. I had to do better. I couldn't just let my own fears, which even my doctors confirmed were unfounded, rule me, my life, and my family as well! I had to do better. I knew that I'd need to reach out more, that I'd need to find a way to do better. Over time, I found that I was making good progress. I was able to drive my kids to school after a while, and after doing so, I'd take my walk that my psychologist friend had prescribed. As silly as it is to admit, that thirty-minute walk every day was fantastic for me. Not only was it healthy for me physically, but it also helped me to mentally decompress as well. It may have been a small effort, but the impact was immense.

Eventually, my wife took a substitute teaching job while I was on disability leave, and I felt that I needed to contribute somehow. I needed to find some way to help out, even if it wasn't working. So, I undertook the bulk of the housework while my wife worked. Cleaning the house and washing dishes helped me feel a bit more structured, responsible, and needed. It made me feel more in control of the environment that I was in. If something in the home was stressing me out, I knew that I could address it. I knew that I would be able to resolve it, that I could change things so that the stress was no longer there.

At the end of my day, I would sit down and write in my journal, also prescribed by my psychologist, and I'd reflect upon the current day. My day would come to an end, and as always, my domestic life continued. Day in and day out was the same. It wasn't exciting, but I settled in. I needed to find something to cling to, and this offered me that chance. But I would not be truthful if I said that I didn't need something to change.

A Step Forward to Socialization

My wife eventually suggested that I get involved in my boys' extracurricular activities. She pushed me to get involved in the

Boy Scouts with them. For her sake, but to my surprise, I eventually became the Cub Master of the Pack. I was leading the children and their activities! I hadn't ever given such a task much thought, but I jumped in head-on. I was actually a bit excited about it, though the anxious part of my mind still filled me with apprehension. I settled in well, though, and I found that I was doing so much better.

Being a Cub Master gave me the opportunity to schedule activities. I was required to attend them too, and that was the best part. I got to enjoy that special time with my boys, watching them as they grow. I found it exciting to watch the sheer joy on the faces of my boys and their Pack. They were happy, the other kids were happy, and I started to realize that I was also feeling happy. Through the anxiety and depression, I finally got that first taste of normalcy, that first bit of happiness that I knew was out there if I tried to reach out for it. I found that I wasn't broken—that I could feel happiness just like anyone else if I reached out, and the Boy Scouts became that source for me.

The privilege of being able to watch over my boys as they launched their water rockets together was immense. The excitement they had over racing pinewood race cars was almost palpable. I found myself actually starting to feel happier and happier. I looked forward to the times we met. I reveled in being able to plan out all of those activities that my boys and their friends would love. It was great being able to think about something as innocent as what kind of activity to do next for the children. It was a well-needed reprieve from the anxiety that I had been living through, and even for a short period of time, I was able to achieve it.

Boy Scouting was good for me in other ways, too. I found that I exercise more often. We went hiking and camping regularly, and that meant that I had to get up and be physical, something that my psychologist had recommended long before I had joined the Boy Scouts. He was right. As my physical shape returned, I felt like I was getting more in touch with my mental health as well. I felt like I was starting to feel a bit better. It was the first push into regular socialization. I needed it to help me create that cozy world that I lived in. If I wanted to be happy, I knew that I had to take charge. I could control some things, and how often I socialize is just one of those elements. If socialization brings me happiness, then I could make it work. I owed it to myself, and I'd find a way to make it work for me.

One way I tried to connect with my community was through attending prayer at the mosque. This was something that I had done before. I was always good about maintaining my worship, and I had religious friends that I'd speak to from time to time to try to make sense of such a strange, difficult, and mysterious world that surrounds us. What once brought me comfort, though, quickly became a source of negativity for me. I found that I wasn't actually as comforted by being at the mosque as I had originally been. It became a daily struggle for me to maintain that consistent worship. I felt obligated to do so, but the more that I attended, the worse I started to feel.

For me, the prayer started to become negative. Some days, I found that I felt even worse than I had felt when I first arrived at the mosque. I was concerned with the focus on hellfire and punishment for nonbelievers. It felt over-the-top, almost too negative, and I found myself really grappling with it. I found that it was really difficult to accept that some people would be punished for their beliefs to the point of spending time burning in Hell.

Yes, I know that this is par for the course in many different religions, but for some reason, I really struggled with it. I didn't like the imagery of death and pain. It was too reminiscent of what I feared—that my own death was seemingly imminent. It left me wondering about how to feel and what I could do to ensure that I was still worshipping and connecting to my religion without making my anxiety worse. It was a delicate balance, especially because I *wanted* to socialize. I wanted to get out of the house. Connecting with my peers and with those who share my faith was something I craved.

Though sometimes I felt like I wanted to, I never quit attending worship. I'd take breaks sometimes when things got too rough or when I felt like my mental health was taking a hit, but I tried hard to stay true to my faith. I didn't want to abandon the religion entirely; I just wanted to be free of that visual image of pain and suffering for others that was bringing me down. I didn't want to think of death. I wanted to go to the mosque to feel at ease, at home, and with those I loved.

Remember, you can't change the environment that you are in, but you can change your position in it. I took that to heart. While I knew that I wouldn't quit my religion, I also knew that there were other options for me. I wanted to keep my community close to me, and I wanted to make sure that I felt that sense of connection that I strove to achieve. I always went back to my place of worship.

For me, I found that despite the hellfire imagery, I could bring myself to find peace in other ways. I could help myself reconnect to my religion by making sure that I felt more involved. I listened to classical music often. I found myself working to find peace for my soul through the lilting melodies, the complex harmonies, and the beautiful sounds of the music that I listened to. It brought me to a point of peace, a point at which I felt like I was comfortable. I was able to reconnect to that love that I desired in order to find a way to soothe my aching soul.

I also chose to work on Quranic recitations and using Islamic prayer beads as I praised Allah (God the Almighty). This helped me to escape the doom and hellfire imagery, allowing me to focus on passages and imagery that I chose myself. It helped me to find peace, to find that connection to my religion, and to feel like I was in more control.

These two simple habits might sound silly to you, but for me, they were lifelines. They helped me to maintain a sense of control and normalcy. They helped me stay on track with what I needed to do to help me feel a bit more capable of dealing with everything that was on my proverbial plate.

Resultantly, my daily habits came together to create my own cozy world, my own reprieve from anxiety and depression. They came together to create some semblance of happiness and peace that I could eventually achieve if I knew what I was doing. I took the little habits at first, building upon them and starting to do one thing after another. Those habits became the foundation that I would use, my springboard to help me to finally make that real progress that I wanted a reality.

Then I started moving toward my ability to socialize with others. I focused on being able to look forward to being around people more often. I knew that I'd be able to find more happiness with them, and they really helped my situation. Boy Scouts gave me that semblance of happiness that I had been looking for. I could see that door to recovery getting closer, little by little. I knew that I was taking the right steps toward finding the freedom of reaching out for that doorknob and opening it. I kept taking those baby steps, but I could see the progress that I was making as I did so, and that was a great motivation for me. Finally, I realized that I could get myself back into attending the mosque, even if I took breaks every now and then. I taught myself that I'd be able to do this, that I could do better, and that I'd be able to find my own happiness by staying true to myself.

Through these three little baby step sequences, I started to create my own cozy world that I knew I would need if I wanted to find my happiness as well. It would be there for me if I reached out for it; I simply needed to start putting the pieces together so everything else would fall into place. However, when I paused and realized how far I had gone, I could see the outline of my progress. I could see that I'd take two steps forward and sometimes meander around, or even take a step back, but that was also alright. I was making progress, and that's what mattered the most. I would remind myself that I was taking those needed baby steps, and that was all I needed to do. I would get there in my own time, gradually, patiently, one small baby step at a time with determination, and that was alright.

Chapter 8: The Blending Approach

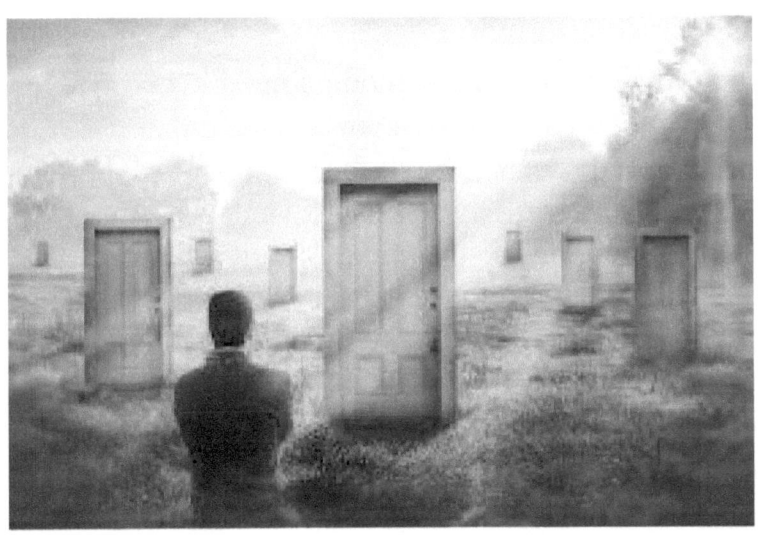

I've never been the kind of person who enjoyed medicine. I always chose to avoid taking any form of aspirin when I had a headache if I knew I had another option to alleviate it. After all, why bother if I could just sleep it off the natural way? I avoided it whenever I could. Even now, I've found that I'm always hesitant to take my anti-anxiety medication. I find it incredibly useful when I find myself on the verge of losing my fight to anxiety, but for the most part, it is a last-ditch effort to keep that anxiety at bay.

When I take my medications, I find myself calming down, but they also usually put me to sleep, which is not very productive if I have a full day ahead of me. I knew that while those medications made for a fantastic sort of lifeline to keep myself free from the throes of my anxiety, I also knew that I would need something that was going to allow me to function as well. I knew that my anxiety was getting worse, but I also knew that I couldn't take the medication every time. I asked my psychiatrist to lower the dosage, and he obliged, prescribing the lowest medication option available. Over time, however, I found myself breaking pills into halves, and sometimes even quarters.

I didn't want to live my life medicated and unable to keep my eyes open. I wanted to handle my affairs my own way, and that motivated me to attempt to use as little of the medication as possible to help myself get through each day. Eventually, I must have gotten something right because I found myself feeling better. I eventually found myself feeling like I was not only able to do better for myself, but as if I wanted to take my newfound happiness and begin spreading it to others as well.

Initiating a New Challenge

I found myself volunteering for the Spiritual Service of Stanford Hospital, as my anxiety became easier to tame. I took the time that I had to go and support patients who were sick. Many of these patients didn't have family members alongside them during their difficult journey. They were all alone in the hospital and in need of a morale boost. No one should have to fight their illnesses alone, nor should they have to recover alone. I knew just how much it meant to me to have my own family there when I needed help, and I felt like the least I could do was help others as well.

So, off I went to do my spiritual duty at Stanford. I'd help them to get through some of the toughest times of their lives. Primarily, I wanted to help people who were Muslim, people whom I could relate to better. We would be able to connect over our faith. But inadvertently, I found myself visiting patients from different religions. Honestly, though I was a bit nervous at first, it ended up being incredibly enriching.

The best experience that I had was the time I found myself in the room of a Russian lady who had just had knee replacement surgery. She was *hilarious*. We might not have shared a bond of the same religion, but really, we're all people of one humanity. We still had plenty to talk about. I got to talk to her about my own experience with a very similar surgery that I went through. We discussed what she had to expect in her future, as well as what my own experiences were. I could tell that she appreciated it, and even though I couldn't give her that spiritual comfort that I tended to give Muslims. I would leave her laughing and laughing about the things that I told her. She loved my stories and was interested in how I am doing now. That experience taught me that I wanted to spend time with people of other faiths as well as with those of my own. I didn't want to limit myself to just Muslim patients—after all, other people would need help as well.

The biggest challenge that I endured, however, was when I was asked to visit the terminally ill patients. It was tough for me to sit there with people who may know that they are dying. I didn't want to give them false hope that they would be just fine in life if they knew that death was imminent. It was a hard line to tow. I'm sure I gave those people hope that they'd get through their condition and that they'd be able to overcome their illnesses and get by just fine. But in a sense, that was almost cruel. I knew that I couldn't continue doing that. I found myself thinking about that situation more and more. I found myself telling myself that *I* could do better. With some introspection, I found myself finding a solution—instead of giving hope to people who were at the point of their bodies giving out, I found myself instead switching to a message of comfort and tranquility. While I needed to know that I wasn't dying to get through my own life, what other people needed to know was that they would be comfortable. I passed along messages of comfort and calmness to people in their final moments in this world. My goal went from cheering people up and giving them hope to understanding that this, too, is a part of life and that it is not totally bad. My new plan worked, and I found myself giving these people the greatest gift that I could: peace of mind as they passed away.

A Setback

When you are younger or middle-aged, you don't expect life to bring you down. You have the idea that **living is** just a given, but the truth is, life is exceedingly fleeting. I feared that with my own anxiety, I was convinced that my demise was impending until my doctor was able to convince me otherwise. I eventually came to the conclusion that death was not imminent and that I'd be just fine in surviving. Of course, I naturally thought the same about most other people as well. I didn't think that we would have a problem losing any friends when we were all still, for all intents and purposes, quite young.

Of course, life has a funny way of testing us when we least expect it, too. It likes to throw curveballs at us that seem almost insurmountable in the face of reality. It likes to take the progress gained and knock you down a few pegs, just to remind you that nothing in life is guaranteed, and to show you just where you are. I faced that test, and it hit me like a ton of bricks. Just when things were becoming normal again, I found that I would need to rely on my focus and strength, and everything that I had been working toward was put to the ultimate test as a direct result of what had happened to me.

My best friend died from hip surgery. I was disappointed that it had happened. He was only in his late forties and quite athletic. In fact, he had injured his hip while playing soccer. He had always been a picture of good health, and when he went in for surgery, we all thought he would be fine. Of course, when someone goes into surgery, there are those concerns, but when it's someone younger and able-bodied, then there are usually fewer concerns **about** what will happen. Of course, when he passed, we were all in shock and were all unable to wrap our minds around what had just happened. It didn't seem real at the moment.

My God, to say that that was a setback was an understatement of the century.

Supporting his family emotionally while I myself desperately wanted some support to keep myself from spiraling was difficult. I needed help with maintaining myself and my own sanity, but that was difficult to manage. After all, his family would get that additional support before I did. It was my duty as his best friend to support his family. I was devastated, but I also understood that I had my role to play, and I was determined to do so.

Though I know that I wasn't ready to hear the news that my friend was gone, it seemed that my valuable time spent volunteering with the hospital left me more equipped to handle such suffering. I realized that I wasn't going to lose myself in this loss. I was more tempered than ever, and that tempering of my personality helped me a lot. Even when I was faced with some of the worst news that I had experienced at that time, I could persevere.

They say that we learn more about ourselves during the hardest times than when everything is fine. It is when we can persevere when we are faced with setbacks that we begin to see how much we have grown as people, and that we can trust who and what we are becoming. I could see this clearly. Even in the darkness of my best friend's death, I could see that I had grown. I was stronger. I could survive taking a hit that I wouldn't have previously been able to endure.

A Major Challenge

As I suffered through some of the most trying times in my life, the idea that I'd go back to work was one that I never doubted. It seemed like a given, I would stay home, recover, and eventually get back to life as it used to be. I was comfortable in my career, and I didn't really want to let that go, though I knew that it brought with it the requirement for travel, especially on air flights. I was torn about that. I knew that I wasn't ready to fly, but I also figured that they would be able to accommodate me with what I needed to do for my own job. But, I tried not to worry about it too much as I got through life. I didn't really think much about the fact that I would have to go back to work or that there was the potential to *not* go back at all. After all, I'd need to support my family, and that meant working.

Eventually, my paid leave of absence ended, and the time to go back to work had arrived. It almost felt sooner than I thought. However, I felt better, and I was ready to face my daily tasks. I was more confident in myself, and I was much more capable of handling my anxiety and depression. I knew that I was able to do so. And yet I still knew that I wasn't ready to fly in airplanes again. I tried to negotiate a different departure or accommodation that would allow me to avoid flying in airplanes when I knew that I wasn't ready yet. But, unfortunately, despite discussions with Human Rights (HR), it didn't work out. There were no other options available to me, and ultimately, I was laid off. I found myself unemployed because of my anxiety and depression, which held me back from air travel.

I should have been upset. I should have been *furious*. But instead, despite knowing that my feelings should have been harsher than they were, I found myself actually feeling *relieved*. There was a huge weight lifted from my shoulders when I realized that I didn't have to continue working there. I wouldn't have to fly again if I didn't want to, and that was a freeing realization. For the first time in a long while, I realized that I had a whole multitude of options available to me. I just had to choose which path I wanted to pursue.

I could have chosen to find a similar job as well, or I could have found something completely new. One decision that I eventually considered was pursuing a complete career change. So, I chose to go back to school to get my Ph.D. In particular, I studied organizational management with the blessing of my wife. She supported me the entire time while I was in school and while I studied. With her support, I was able to become a full-time student. I dedicated myself to my studies more than anything else, next to my family. I was determined and driven to succeed, and I knew the more that I poured myself into it, the better I would be. I spent four long years studying and researching, and when those years were up, I became a professor.

Again, I had to stop and marvel at the universe. We go through these trials in life. We find ourselves struggling and suffering sometimes, but we can take that struggle and transform it into something better. I realized that even though I was struggling, I was growing. I took the opportunity for success, and I ran for it. I worked to make the best out of a difficult situation and found that it paid off over and over again. I knew that I made the right choice in going back to school, and so far, I have not regretted it in the least. It was difficult, but what doesn't kill you makes you stronger, and I have chosen to live by that motto over and over again.

Chapter 9: The Secret Ingredient

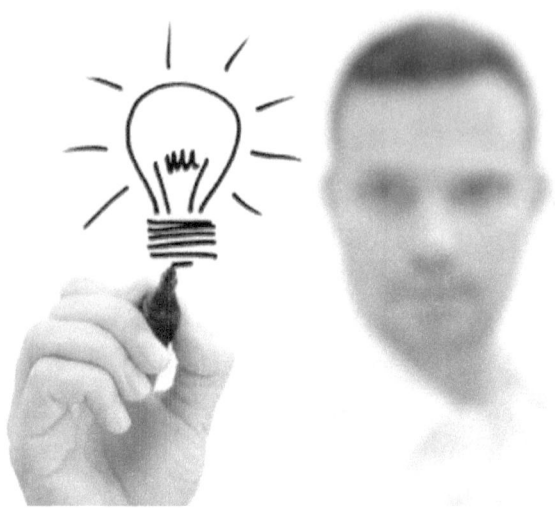

When you read self-help books that promise to solve all of your problems if you only pay attention to what they are offering you and apply the information to yourself so that you can be certain to use it, you realize that the advice is quite similar. You have the energy to remember to be positive when you are stuck facing struggles and other similar situations. They instruct you to look toward the future and to take life one step at a time. They also suggest that ultimately, you are the only one responsible for yourself and your reactions, which, apart from family support, is true. However, that doesn't help very much when you're in the midst of a panic attack.

One thing that I found interesting was that if we are all responsible for our own actions and reactions, why is it that all of the self-help books state that you should surround yourself with positive people? They say that you are the sum of the five people that you interact with the most, and honestly, I've found that to be true. I've applied this concept to my life, and it is no coincidence that I am surrounded by such supportive people in my life. I've chosen who

I wanted to be around carefully. They may not be perfect people, but who is? They are just right for me. They are exactly who I want in my life, and they are here for a reason.

I've chosen to surround myself with people who are just like me, but they still manage to ignite my passion for learning and growing. They are there to make me into a better person, and I see them as the treasures that they are. I know that I have them to rely on. I know that I can look to them and trust that they'll have my back when I need them the most. They are my source of inspiration throughout life, and I know that whenever I need advice, there is bound to be someone in my circle whom I can turn to. And, when it came time for me to get another hint of the recovery that I could have, my fifth lifesaver came from that circle of people that I chose to surround myself with.

The Beautiful Mind

One of my friends, A.Z., was an inspiring fellow. He was an MD with a Sufi character. He was incredibly creative and even almost artistic. His attempts to treat other people involved his own personal touch of blending the science of medicine with spiritual advice as well. He was skilled at finding that point where they intersected, and he worked to provide the best for his patients. He wanted to make sure that they got a holistic approach to their treatment, recognizing that they would need to be treated both in body and mind. He was a curious fellow, and I genuinely enjoyed it when we got to meet together.

At one such meeting, he took the time to speak to me. He was interested in how I was doing. He wanted to make sure that I was able to be healthy, and he cared about my general well-being. In typical A.Z. fashion, he had his own nontraditional recommendations, and on a day that I met with him, he recommended to me that I watch a movie called "The Beautiful Mind." I watched it at his request, and to my surprise, I understood it. I understood why he was suggesting it to me, and I was more than interested in figuring out how to apply it to what I had to do with myself.

The film was about American mathematician John Nash. Dr. Nash was incredibly gifted and intelligent. He was even invited to the Pentagon to aid in cracking encrypted telecommunications from the enemy, which was done with ease. He was smart and constantly looking for more than his usual duties at MIT, including being a teacher. He eventually fell in love with one of his students, and they married. Throughout the film, he is being asked to help thwart a Soviet plot, and it eventually culminates in him believing that he is running away from Soviet agents, who are actually psychiatrists trying to treat him. He is eventually diagnosed with paranoid schizophrenia, and it turns out the person who was trying to get him to help with the Soviet plot was actually a part of his schizophrenia. He eventually learns to overcome his hallucinations, learning to ignore them rather than allow them to rule his life. He eventually manages to teach again and wins the Nobel Prize for his work on Game Theory. He never stopped having hallucinations, but he did learn how he could ignore them and remove their power over him.

He adapted to his schizophrenia and became immensely successful. He didn't let his own mental illness hold him down. He was able to live with those images, to allow them to exist, while he, too, coexisted with them. This movie resonated with me. Now, I wasn't schizophrenic, but I was suffering from major depression. I found myself thinking about the story and the moral within it. I could see exactly why my friend recommended that I watch the movie, and I felt like it did me a lot of good to see it being applied to me. I felt stronger seeing what the movie showed me, and I wanted to apply the same concepts to my own life.

I started to wonder how I could cope with my own depression. The words of my psychologist echoed in my mind as I tried to find the answer: "Either you ignore it, or you find the cause of it." That sounded easier said than done. I couldn't ignore it. Depression was there so intensely that it was impossible to ignore. I couldn't find the cause of it either, or I wasn't sure why I had it. I also wasn't sure what made me the way that I was. It was a question I had pondered long before that point, but was never able to define. I eventually came to the conclusion that I would need to be like Dr. Nash. It was time to stop following the conventional approach and make my own way. I would need my own personal recipe if I wanted to be successful, and I was determined to find out how to make it work for me as well.

I started to reread my journal. I went back and really read it, paying attention to all of the small details. I read not only the words as they were written but also the undertones that existed there as well. I was writing my thoughts and feelings, but there were patterns there, just waiting to be uncovered. I had things to learn, patterns to discern, and hints toward solving my problem, all written there. I looked at what I had gained over those last four years. There were times that were awful. Times when I was certain that I would break, where nothing seemed worth it, and I was certain that I would die.
There were times when I felt like nothing I did would ever be good enough, and that I would never be able to succeed. I thought that I was a waste and a burden, and I could see that in my writing.

But there were good times as well. I could see that through my writing, things weren't as bad as I thought they were at the moment. I could see that I was convinced things were terrible, but

I could also see that I also saw things from the point of bias. I could see that my own thoughts had changed and evolved over the years. I no longer thought of things in that fractured pattern, where every bad was horrible, and every good was an exception to the rule. I felt like back then, when I was really stuck in my depression, that it was impossible for me to get through life because I had that fractured view. I kept wanting to see things independently of each other, but all things that happen are connected. Everything flows, and as I have grown older and wiser, I've discovered this to be the case. I've chosen to look at the world as a sort of comprehensive entity. My world view is all about looking at it as a whole. I chose to see the bad with the good, and as they are related to each other. When you are able to look at them together, you realize that life isn't so bad.

I found that when I was terrified that I would die, I was more interested in listening. I would find myself moved immensely by what other people have to say. I was incredibly empathetic, and I wanted to share their concerns. I would put my heart into my interactions with people, even if those conversations were not. I'm one of those people who will go around and absorb the emotions of other people. I feel like I take on their feelings as if they were my own. I feel their pain passionately, and I find myself driven by the fact that I can relate to them. I think it's tough at times, and I want more than ever to be remembered as a loving person, but during those darkest years of my life, I felt like I was a source of pain. I felt as if I would leave those that I loved with scars as I passed through their lives.

But I realized something: even if I bring other people pain, as they bring to me as well sometimes, we can also enjoy each other's happiness. I can share the concerns of my loved ones, and while they are close to my heart and therefore able to hurt me more intensely than anyone else in my life, we can share our joy, and that is where we ought to be. That realization that I could tap into my empathetic feelings with others was what mattered more than anything else to me.

Again, I found myself realizing that the best good in life comes from being able to connect to others, and through my grapple with depression and feeling like my own life was going to be ripped away from me in the blink of an eye, I realized something important: I can do better. I can be better. I can be the person that I wanted to be, and I can ensure that I am more than I thought I was. Once again, I realized that the best of life comes from the worst, and through the darkness, I found that I shone brightly.

I would not have this realization, this understanding that we are so closely connected and that we can bring each other this contentment if it weren't for my depression. It might sound strange, but my bout with depression actually taught me to reflect. It taught me to reflect more on my experiences as I have them. It also taught me to reflect closely on the world around me, and on my life and the experiences that I've had. It has taught me to realize that through listening carefully to those around us, I could overcome any obstacle.

I came to appreciate my depression and the lessons that it taught me in life. It became like any other difficult situation that I had to overcome. It taught me those important lessons in my life that I never knew I needed, and it was not as bad as I thought. Just like I could not become the scholar that I am without the rigorous training from my Ph.D. studies, I needed my depression to teach me to become the kind, empathetic individual that I am today. In my Ph.D. program, I learned to shape my mind. I worked through reading, through writing, through learning to take criticism and give my own feedback to others. I had to make certain that my mind was nimble and that I was creative in approaching the challenges that I had to face. My Ph.D. helped my mind to flourish and blossom to its fullest potential.

While my Ph.D. shaped my mind, I know that my depression shaped my heart. It was not easy. It hurt. It showed me that there is very real darkness in the world, but through that darkness, I began to see the truth. I saw that people matter and that I have a support system that cares about me. I recognized that I had people in my life who loved me, who wanted me to get better. I had friends and family all rally around me, and I honestly do believe that I would not be the successful man that I am today without my experiences. My depression, those four years that I thought would break me down, was actually the incubator that my heart needed. Just like a caterpillar must break down within its chrysalis to become a butterfly, I felt like my heart broke down to be transformed as well.

My appreciation for depression has overcome my fears of it. I'm no longer afraid because I see the truth. I know that depression is there, and I still can respect that I was afraid at that time. It was terrifying to feel like I was going to die. It was a horrible feeling to be weighed down, to feel like I was being drowned or smothered by my mind. But, over time, I became almost immune to the feeling of being down. I realized that I could work beyond those feelings, that they didn't have that same control over me as they used to. I knew that the feelings were still there, and I knew that depression was still there, but I was also able to defeat that control. It wasn't able to control me any longer because I was able to appreciate the lessons that it brought me, and I realized that it wasn't as bad. Life wasn't as bad. My thoughts weren't as bad.

The new mindset that I took and the perception shift in the world were a great step toward my recovery from depression. It was slow progress. It took time for me to begin to get better, and it took time for me to even realize that I was improving. But, as time passed, I eventually realized that my anxiety attacks were beginning to steadily decrease. Even when I did experience anxiety, I could tell that they weren't as severe. If I had a full-blown panic attack, I would be able to overcome it, and sometimes, all I really needed was half a pill of my medicine, and I was able to continue working like usual.

Like Dr. Nash, I came up with my own ways of coping. I knew that I was not trying to defeat the anxiety and depression, but rather I was trying to live alongside them. I was working for coexistence over anything else, and when I adjusted my goalposts accordingly, I realized that it was far easier for me to cope. I didn't have to be perfect. My mind didn't have to be perfect. It just had to work for me, and when I could get to that point, I knew that I'd be just fine. I realized that recovery was within my grasp and that I'd be able to live a normal life.

The door to my freedom was within my reach. It was so close that I could feel it. I was able to reach for it, to wrap my fingers around the proverbial knob and open it up. I found that the world on the other side was a beautiful one, and it was almost brighter due to the time I spent in the darkness, and for that, I could find a real appreciation.

Time for the Goodbye

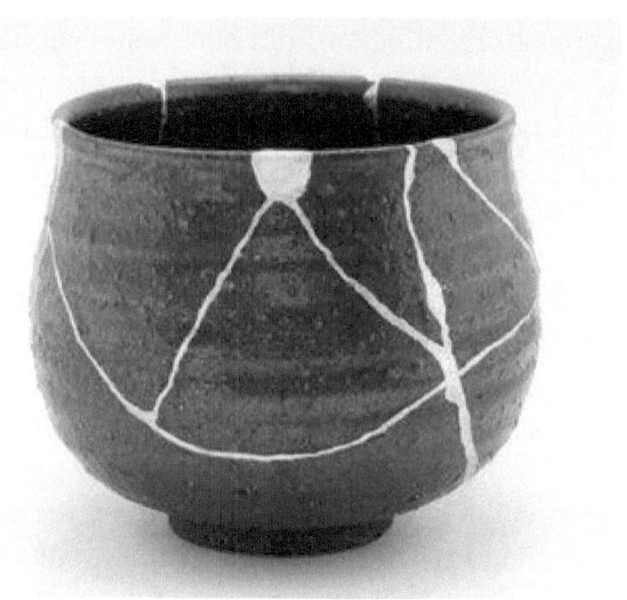

As I found myself becoming more and more capable of coping with my feelings, life didn't seem as difficult. I could see the good in the world, something that my depression had convinced me to ignore. The good thing is there you just have to open your eyes to see it.

I had coffee with a good friend, J.D., one day. As we were sitting at a table and speaking, he asked me how I was doing. He was curious about how my anxiety attacks had been going and whether they were still as bad. I could tell he was worried. I smiled at him and informed him that they were getting better. I knew that I'd be able to live with them without too much of a problem. They weren't overwhelming or anything. I was getting better every day. I was growing stronger.

He prodded a bit deeper. He asked how I was doing with my depression. I knew he was a concerned friend, and I was glad that he was. The fact that he cared so much made me feel like I was loved and supported. But I also wanted him to know that I was different. The depression had changed me indelibly—it had left its mark on me, and I needed to get that point across to him.

I took a piece of paper and drew a long line on it. The graphite left a thick, dark mark across the surface. Then I flipped my pencil over and erased it as my friend watched with polite curiosity. I rubbed away the line to the best of my ability, but there was still a shadow of the mark left on the paper. It would always be there—there was no way for me to get it all off completely. I handed the piece of paper to him and asked: "Do you think that this paper is the same as it was before I drew the line and erased it?" "No," he conceded after a moment of hesitation. He looked down at the paper long and hard.

I agreed with him. There was no way around it. The paper had been permanently traced and marked by my pencil. I told him that in the same way that my pencil had marked my paper, the depression had marked me. There were still traces of it within me, and they may always be there. I was not the same person I was before. I had changed greatly during my time between where I was before and where I was at that point. My depression changed me. It left my soul feeling a bit more fragile, but still whole. I had more depth, more wisdom, and more experience. I was still me, but I was wiser. I wasn't ashamed of my depression, and it wasn't like a scar that I had to hide. Just as the faint pencil line remained on the paper after it was erased, it left a mark, a fingerprint on my soul, but that mark taught me a lot about myself, my destiny, and my life.

The ancient Japanese art of Kintsugi is a wonderful lesson that I can relate to. A story goes that a 15th-century military commander broke the tea bowl that he loved. He wanted it to be repaired, but he didn't want it to be married. Instead, the repair was done with gold. Kintsugi became a way that broken dishes were repaired, with the seams treated with lacquer and gold. The final product didn't try to hide the break in the material, but rather it made it better. It became a way to celebrate the notion that despite the rough edges, despite the challenges, and despite the times when we all fall apart, we can be put back together again, and the final product can be that much more beautiful than what it had been previously. Depression was like that—it was those cracks that had to be repaired over time, but I am now so much more, a person, and so much better than I was before. I have persevered, and I have come out on the other dark side, someone that I am proud to be.

Whoever and wherever you are, please know that depression is only a monster if you regard it that way. Depression hurts. It is hard to bear. It lies to you and tries to convince you that you are at your worst. It wants you to believe all of those things and that you are worthless, or that nothing will ever be the same, and the truth is, they won't be. But they will not always be hopeless. They will not always be painful. They will not always leave in despair and wonder if there is any reason to try to get better.

If you have depression, then it will be an opportunity for you to make the most out of a negative situation. It is there to teach you that you can discover your inner self. It helps you to see the world around you in a better light, with the wisdom of someone who has suffered the way that you have suffered. The symptoms may be there far longer than you would like, and they may take far longer than you wish to go away, but the truth is, you can do it. You can come out on top in this situation. You can overcome it, and you can be better when you do. Your own heart may be laying in pieces right now, but you can put it back together, bit by bit, binding them together with a kind of Kintsugi gold, and you will find that you will become a much more radiant person when you are done.

Remember, depression develops slowly. The symptoms build up over time, and that means that it will take time for them to dissipate as well. Don't try to rush back into normalcy before you are ready. Take the time to get to know yourself. Learn the lessons that your depression has in store for you and figure out what it will take for you to overcome it. It will be there until you do something to change, and ultimately, only you have that power.

It is only when you learn those lessons and begin to understand what you can do with yourself that you can then begin to move forward. You can tell yourself that you are done with it, you can remind yourself that you are ready to move on. You will eventually be able to reach out, open the door to normalcy, and find your way back into a fruitful life again. When you get there, you'll have the opportunity that I did.

As I sat there in the café with my friend J.D., I realized that I was closing that chapter in my life. I was there, looking back at everything I had overcome. My hand was still on the proverbial doorknob that I had been striving for, and all I had to do was turn it, step out, and close it forever. All I had to do was make that choice. I chose to do so, and I walked away from it. I closed the door that led to the darkness behind me. I had learned my lessons. I had grown as a person. I had a newfound appreciation for the world and for life, and with those lessons within me and my newfound respect for my struggles, I realized that I was exactly where I was meant to be in life. As the door shut on that chapter of my story, I found myself feeling lighter. I could finally say what I had been hoping to say for four agonizing years, and what you will be able to say when you are ready.

Goodbye, Depression.

I extend my very best wishes and appreciation to all those who stood by me and helped through my agonizing experiences, and for that, I shall be eternally grateful.

Magdy Hussein, Ph.D.

www.ingramcontent.com/pod-product-compliance
Lightning Source LLC
Chambersburg PA
CBHW020600220526
45463CB00006B/2390